Gay Men's Literature in the Twentieth Century

MARK LILLY

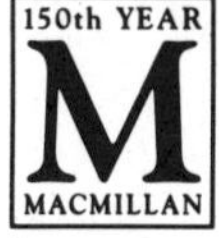

First published 1993 by
THE MACMILLAN PRESS LTD
Houndmills, Basingstoke, Hampshire RG21 2XS
and London
Companies and representatives
throughout the world

A catalogue record for this book is available
from the British Library.

ISBN 0–333–49435–0 hardcover
ISBN 0–333–49436–9 paperback

Typeset by Nick Allen/Longworth Editorial Services
Longworth, Oxon.

Printed in Hong Kong

This book is dedicated to all those militant activists in the lesbian and gay community whose courage and tenacity in the face of overwhelming odds is an inspiration to us all. If Britain ever becomes a civilised and just society, it will partly be as a result of their selfless efforts.

Contents

Acknowledgements

The author and publishers wish to thank the following for permission to use copyright material:

Rosica Colin Ltd., on behalf of the author's Estate for the extracts from 'Reserve' and 'Soliloquy 1' in *Collected Poems* by Richard Aldington. Copyright © 1948, 1976 Richard Aldington.

Faber and Faber Ltd., for the extract from 'The Modern Achilles' in *The Buried Stream* by Geoffrey Faber, 1941.

David Higham Associates Ltd., on behalf of the author's Estate for the extract from 'My Company' in *Collected Poems* by Herbert Read (Faber and Faber).

Macmillan Publishers Ltd., for the extracts from 'Lament' in *Whin* by Wilfrid Gibson and 'Sentry Go' in *Neighbours* by Wilfrid Gibson.

Random Century Group, for the extract from 'Fulfilment' in *Ardours and Endurances* by Robert Nicholls (Chatto & Windus), and 'The Secret' by Robert Nicholls in *Aurelia and Other Poems* (Chatto & Windus).

Every effort has been made to trace all the copyright holders, but if any have been inadvertently overlooked the publisher will be pleased to make the necessary arrangement at the first opportunity.

I was greatly assisted in my work by previous studies, notably Greg Woods's *Articulate Flesh,* Martin Taylor's anthology of First World War poetry, *Lads,* with its fine introduction; and Henry Scott Stokes's *The Life and Death of Yukio Mishima*. I thank these authors warmly for their assistance. Particular thanks are also due to Robert Rebein, of the University of Buffalo, who made detailed suggestions for changes and additions.

Introduction

In an ecstasy of incoherent rage, his father proceeded to spit repeatedly on the pages until his chin was covered with saliva; then he lifted the book to his mouth, and dismembered it with his teeth. When his innocent son bravely persisted in demanding what it was that Oscar Wilde had done, he received the answer written on a scrap of paper: Illum crimen horribile . . . quod non nominandum est. [*That horrible crime . . . which is not to be named.*]

(Beverley Nichols being caught reading *Dorian Gray*)

. . . all a piece of literature should do, I think, is tell you what it was like touching Frank Romero's lips for the first time on a hot afternoon in August in the bathroom of Les's Café on the way to Fire Island.

(Andrew Holleran, *Dancer from the Dance*)

Poet, you are no liar. The world that you imagine
is the real one. The melodies of the harp
alone know truth, and in this life
they can be our only true guides.

(Cavafy, 'The Poet and the Muse')

. . . the great difference between people in this world is not between the rich and the poor or the good and the evil, the biggest of differences in this world is between the ones that had or have pleasure in love and those that haven't and hadn't any pleasure in love, but just watched it with envy, sick envy.

(Tennessee Williams, *Sweet Bird of Youth*)

His life, passions, trials, loves, were, at worst, filth, and, at best, disease in the eyes of the world, and crimes in the eyes of his countrymen. There were no standards for him except those he could make for himself. There were no standards for him because he could not accept the definitions, the hideously mechanical jargon of the age. He saw no one around him worth his envy, did not believe in the vast, grey sleep which was called security, did not believe in the cures, panaceas, and slogans which afflicted the world he knew; and this meant that he had to create his standards and make up his definitions as he went along. It was up to him to find out who he was, and it was his necessity to do this . . . alone.

(James Baldwin, *Another Country*)

I don't know if you're living still
Or fallen in the fight
But in my heart your heart is safe
Till the last night
(First World War poem, 'His Mate', by Studdert Kennedy)

All of these extracts appear in this book. Seen together, they give an idea of the extraordinary diversity of approach amongst the writers I propose to discuss. Tenderness lies side by side with rage, existential rejection of conventions rubs shoulders with sexual hedonism. Only with steady reflection can we tease out some shared preoccupations.

Each chapter in this book is dedicated to the work of an author who was or is predominantly or exclusively gay, with the exception of the chapter on the poetry of the First World War (the reasons for making the exception are set out in the chapter itself) and the section on Byron (who was bisexual). The book is an introduction, and has been written with the first-year college and university student, and the general reader, especially in mind. It would of course be gratifying to find my academic colleagues amongst its readers, but it is not designed for them. I have tried to do without most of the technical jargon of academic criticism, and to write as clearly and concisely as possible. Clarity of exposition has been my guiding principle.

For the most part, each chapter deals with a single author. I have written each of the separate chapters in such a way that each one forms part of a continuing argument about gay writing across the whole period, but also so that each chapter makes sense as a separate essay. This is because there will be readers who have an interest in one or two authors, but do not wish to work their way through the whole book.

This book is not a general survey, and therefore in the selection of authors for discussion, I have made no attempt to be comprehensive. There is, for example, nothing on major figures like Proust, Gide, Mann or Auden, or on contemporary writers who have attracted considerable acclaim such as Thom Gunn, Edmund White and Agustin Gomez-Arcos. Instead, my aim has been to choose a limited number of texts from a limited number of writers in order to investigate certain shared themes and patterns. Confining the scope in this way has allowed me to give detailed readings of individual texts, in a way that is impossible in a general survey. Of course, my choices are personal and the reader must judge their suitability. Nevertheless, I should like to provide a short rationale for them.

A key principle was coherence; that is, positively to choose a group of gay authors whose work could be discussed in the form, as it were, of a developing story. From Byron onwards, the writers studied here all express a rejection of the society in which they find themselves. They fall into two groups. There are those, following Shakespeare's Coriolanus, who say defiantly, on their expulsion from society, 'There is a world elsewhere' and, when banished, retort, 'I banish you!' Genet, Baldwin and Mishima, in their deep loathing of contemporary society, adopt this attitude, renounce the world vehemently, but combine their vigorous iconoclasm with implied or explicit suggestions for a different world. The second group of writers, people like Forster, Isherwood and Leavitt, are reformers rather than rebels. They speak calmly, trying to move or cajole the reader into tolerant attitudes and a renunciation of prejudice. They want to change a few details here and there rather than sweep the whole board clean.

Within both groups certain themes emerge repeatedly. There is the existentialist determination not to accept social rules and customs for their own sake; each person must have the courage to realise his freedom through exercising it, often in defiance of social norms. Then there is the theme of self-contempt: gay characters (in Baldwin, Holleran and Williams, for example) who accept society's evaluation of their own worth without question, and whose regrettable fate is therefore to be seen as in some sense self-inflicted. Most of these writers also articulate a desire to escape from the oppressive heterosexual world into an alternative one. This might be the crazy drug-drenched excitement of Holleran's discos in New York and Fire Island; or the pastoral idyll in Forster's *Maurice*; or the world of artistic creation in the poetry of Cavafy; or the zany world of 'camp' humour in the plays of Orton. Most of these works examine the notion of the outsider. Societies have a need to identify easy targets – gays, Jews, blacks – for abuse and, if necessary, murder, in order to exorcise their anxieties about their lives, over which they clearly feel they have no control. As these themes emerge again and again in different forms, diversely expressed but nevertheless suggesting a certain cohesion and uniformity, their significance and meaning for the reader of this book will, I hope, be satisfactorily amplified and enriched.

This book is intended as a contribution towards the field of gay studies. In comparison with the established success, especially in the United States, of studies based on women and race, gay studies are in their infancy. The specialist publishing houses, academic sub-committees, university and college courses, grants – in fact the whole apparatus by means of which the world knows that an area of study has arrived at 'respectability' – are not as firmly in place for gay studies as for studies centring on women and people of colour. However, despite the considerable opposition, it looks clear that they will not only continue to develop, but to expand at a dramatic rate. But there is a lively and continuing debate about their rationale. I should like to set out – especially for the benefit of readers new to the debate – some of the questions that are raised by the very existence of gay studies.

We need to start with the question of purpose. Why have gay or black or women's studies at all? Surely they encourage the separatist tendencies of Western culture generally. An intellectual ghetto has the same adverse effects as a physical one: people divided from each other, a kind of informal apartheid. The merit of literary studies under the traditional dispensation, so it is argued, is that, irrespective of considerations of gender, race, sexual orientation or any other defining category, works can be discussed and interpreted using tools of criticism which, because they represent a unifying consensus, also bestow prestige and even reliability on the resulting judgements.

This complaint voices a legitimate concern. Many of those involved in what I propose to call 'minority studies' (to be understood as including women) address it by saying that they like to think of these studies as temporary and provisional, in the way that I suggest below all critical approaches are. The argument runs that, at the present moment, mainstream culture ignores and debases minority experience (this is more fully developed in chapter 1), and therefore in order both to counteract the negative stereotypes and the prejudiced or culturally ill-informed commentaries of the traditionalists, there needs to be a period in which a more or less sustained, committed and concentrated attack takes place. Once the value of minority experience is understood and valued, academic separatism can wither on the vine. However, it is only fair to add that there are more hard-line separatists who cannot imagine heterosexuals ever accommodating themselves to the legitimate aspirations of gay people (and so for men/women; black/white) and we must therefore resign ourselves to an indefinite future in which interest groups exist as openly in the academy as they do in the world of society and politics.

There are three other major complaints made by opponents of gay/black/women's studies. First, intellectual endeavour requires neutrality, but the vast majority of those engaged in such studies are partisans or members of the group involved, and unembarrassedly declare their commitment to advance the status and interests of the group. How can academic studies be impartial if there is a fixed agenda in advance, and certain unfavourable conclusions are likely to be suppressed?

Secondly, minority studies are seen as political in the sense that they seek to destabilise and discredit mainstream assumptions about culture and value. An excellent example of this is taking place as I write (Spring 1991) in Washington DC, where an exhibition of paintings on the theme of the American West has been supplied with a catalogue and commentary interpreting famous canvasses not in the established way (as giving validity and even glory to white Americans' territorial incursions against the Indians) but in a way that castigates those deeds as barbarous.

Thirdly, the traditional criteria of literary excellence are seen to be under threat from minority studies. Novels and poems which, under the old dispensation, would not have been considered (to put it baldly) good enough to be studied, are now being allowed onto syllabuses because of fashion. Furthermore, they are actively displacing some of the great classics which have already proved their worth. Ephemeral works should not be accorded the same status as canonic texts whose survival over time is clear evidence of their excellence. It is not suggested that literary works of minority interest should be omitted from syllabuses; but that their place there should be won not because they are 'relevant' or fashionable, but because they are fine works of art according to the traditional criteria.

We now turn to the arguments of the defence. First, if minority studies are partisan, then so are traditional studies. The difference lies in the fact that the partisanship of the first group is openly avowed and clearly understood, whereas that of the second group constitutes a sort of hidden agenda. Individual traditionalists may not even be fully aware themselves of the nature of their own partisanship, but such lack of awareness does not reduce its effect. Furthermore, it is now an accepted commonplace that 'neutrality' or non-partisanship is impossible; we can and do see things only from a subjective standpoint. Of course, some interpretations are regularly described as being more 'objective' than others, but this is often an impression created by a certain apparently detached linguistic style and does not necessarily reflect a substantive difference.

Secondly, if practitioners of minority studies are to be described as intent on discrediting mainstream cultural values, the answer is a happy acknowledgement that this is indeed the case. It is not clear why such an approach is any different from the vehement *protection* of mainstream cultural values. There are defenders and attackers in any battle, but they are all equally fighters.

The third charge has proved to be the most contentious: that established and tested criteria of excellence are replaced by whimsical fashionable notions of political relevance, with the result that 'inferior' works are studied. The answer to this, put simply, is that there is no justification for assuming that traditional criteria are 'better' than novel ones, or that considerations of, for example, fashion or political concern should be considered inferior to any others. In addition, there is an unacknowledged dishonesty in the traditionalists' case which consists in the implied pretence that the mainstream literary criteria on which they rely have a lengthy historical pedigree. In fact, their critical assumptions are quite modern, and if they were to look only a little backwards they would find much to quarrel with. For example, eighteenth-century writers like Pope, Addison, Steele and Swift took it for granted that literature was, partly at least, political propaganda. In the nineteenth century, an important test of the worthiness of a novel was whether it was fit for ladies and could be left in the drawing-room; *Jane Eyre*, to give one example, was not. We should also look to the future when considering this issue. It is more than likely that at some possibly near date in the future *Moby Dick* will be seen as a wicked book by virtue of its 'speciesism' (it deals with the cruel persecution of a dumb animal) just as it is now considered by feminist criticism as a statement of masculine assertiveness by virtue, *inter alia*, of the almost complete absence of female characters. Literature is read, and can only be read, in the context of societies in which hundreds of variables alter and adjust the way we want to search for value. We should bear in mind that, when we consider the past, every set of critical assumptions and practices since Aristotle now seems to us to be either simplistic, offensive, absurd or at the very least radically incomplete. So it will be with 'new criticism', structuralism, deconstruction; and so it will certainly be with gay studies as a concept. The traditionalists' implied claim to have discovered some transcendent criteria, good for all time, is therefore profoundly unhistorical.

Finally, a word about the term 'gay men's literature'. There is no consensus at the moment as to its scope, and it can therefore include some or all of the following categories: works that deal with homosexuality written by heterosexuals; works by closeted gay men, writing without direct reference to homosexuality, whose meaning is nevertheless informed by the writer's sexuality (Forster's *The Longest Journey*, Tennessee Williams's *The Glass Menagerie*); the work of gay writers seemingly unaware (consciously) of their sexuality, but articulating it nevertheless (the Hopkins of *The Bugler's First Communion* and *Harry Ploughman*); and finally the work of 'out' gay writers, addressing issues of homosexual desire and culture directly (Andrew Holleran, Edmund White).

1

The Homophobic Academy

In the Introduction, in explaining in general terms why there is a need for gay studies, I promised to discuss in detail what mainstream critical practice amounted to over issues of homosexuality in literature, so that the move towards a different approach would be understood. I propose to do that now. I shall discuss the issues of censorship, marginalisation, abuse and critical assumptions in modern literary studies, and conclude with an extended example of homophobic writing in the work of Jeffrey Meyers.

In 1818, Thomas Bowdler published *The Family Shakespeare,* an edition of the plays in which large sections of text had been cut in order to remedy what was thought a terrible defect in an otherwise fine playwright. Bowdler's policy was to omit 'whatever is unfit to be read aloud by a gentleman to a company of ladies'.[1] I cite the case of Dr Bowdler because there are some commentators who point to his *Family Shakespeare* as a self-evident example of the absurdity of all censorship, even as they seek the extension of the blasphemy laws in the wake of the Salman Rushdie affair in order to protect the sensibilities of non-Christian believers, or wish to strengthen legal prohibitions against incitement to racial hatred. There is, of course, a case to be made for saying that Victorian horror at the mention of sex is less worthy of concern than, say, a Christian's horror at the defamation of his God. Much depends on the reasons giving rise to the interdiction. I mention this point so that it will not be thought that I assume all cases of censorship to be automatically wrong. Rather, my purpose here is largely confined to commenting on its nature.

The history of the overt censorship of gay literature, either in society generally or in the various levels of education from schools to universities, is well documented. Popular editions of Auden and Rimbaud omit the overtly gay poems. Romantic fictions studied in schools always centre on heterosexual couples. Questions have been asked in the House of Commons about the novels of David Rees, and one of them[2] was removed from a list of books recommended for use in schools which was compiled by the Inner London Education Authority. London's specialist gay bookshop (Gay's the Word) was raided in the 1980s, and copies of works by Gore Vidal, Jean Genet, Oscar Wilde, Thom Gunn and others were taken away by the authorities for examination. Most recently, in Britain, the effect of the internationally notorious Clause 28 of the Local Government Act 1988 (which prohibits the 'promotion of homosexuality' by local councils) has been such that many councils, such as Avon and Somerset, have as a result instituted a rigorous vetting procedure for public library books that give positive images of lesbian and gay people. Those that defame and insult, such as many of those found in the medical and religious sections of libraries, remain unmolested on the shelves.

In the practice of literary criticism, however, censorship is frequently more subtle than this. Its weapon is more usually omission. John Osborne's review of a typical example of this, Michael Stapleton's *Cambridge Guide to English Literature* (1983), tells much of the story:

> [Adrienne Rich and Radclyffe Hall are omitted.] Robbie Burns' philanderings with a variety of women are sympathetically recorded, but our author can hardly bring himself to mention the subject of homosexuality. Katherine Mansfield's unhappy marriages . . . are chronicled, but not her extended affair with Ida Constance Baker. The entries on Melville, Whitman, Harold Nicolson and Somerset Maugham avoid their homosexual experiences. Gertrude Stein's lifelong devotion to Alice B. Toklas is presented as companionship rather than lesbian love (no chance here that our author will note the sly genital reference in the title of Stein's brilliant *Tender Buttons*). At times such censorship (for that is what it amounts to) is risible in its effects. Hence, our text has the unavoidable distinction of failing to explain why Oscar Wilde was imprisoned, or why E. M. Forster's frankly homoerotic novel *Maurice* was published posthumously. Again, W. H. Auden's marriage to Erika Mann is mentioned, but not that he was a committed homosexual

who entered the contract to give a refugee from the Nazis . . . American citizenship.[3]

Many prestigious critics like Terry Eagleton are found making the now obligatory acknowledgements of the importance in literary criticism of considerations of colour and gender,[4] but say nothing at all about gay perspectives. Fleur Adcock's long and thorough introduction to the *Faber Book of Women's Poetry* contains, despite the presence of distinguished lesbian poets in the collection, not a single mention of lesbian issues. It is not uncommon to see surveys of feminist literature written by feminists, in which lesbian issues are omitted. Most of the works written on Christopher Marlowe's play *Edward the Second* do not even mention its major theme: the love affair between Gaviston and the king. The repeated efforts by Anthony Burgess to scotch the idea that there was 'anything queer' about D. H. Lawrence; and the recent correspondence in the *London Review of Books*[5] from C. K. Stead denouncing a new biography of Katherine Mansfield by Claire Tomalin, because it reveals her lesbian experiences, are recent examples. The idea is the protection of the sacred name: again and again, studies on Wilde, Mann, Proust, Marlowe, Sassoon, Gide omit the homosexual element. Critics are especially nervous about bisexuality; hence the panic when Shakespeare, Tennyson or T. S. Eliot have gay sentiments attributed to their work. As a young undergraduate, my first lecture on T. S. Eliot was given by a lecturer (now a poet), who commented on 'the filthy lie' that Eliot 'loved' Jean Verdenal, the dedicatee of *The Waste Land*. Even in rather out of the way places, such as among the ranks of the A. E. Housman Society, one finds the same sentiment. Members have sterilised Housman of his sexuality, and read the poems as expressions of merely brotherly affection. Often, if not usually, the literary disciple, finding him/herself with two irreconcilable facts (great esteem for the writer; evidence of the latter's homosexuality) simply excludes the second, inconvenient, one from the mind. Many T. E. Lawrence admirers are still claiming that their favourite was a straight-down-the-line heterosexual.

Rather different to the practice of actual censorship is that of marginalisation. In a sense this is more interesting because its meaning and significance is not always understood by those who actually do it. For example, Patricia Hodgart, referring to Plato's

Symposium says, in passing, 'Love, incidentally, in this context is not heterosexual love.'[6] At the heart of Plato's work is an assumption that the love between two men is superior to that existing between a man and a woman, so that the use of the word 'incidentally' seems unaccountable. What we have here, in my view, is not an example of the unscholarly but a sort of half-conscious *embarrassment*. Put simply, the desire not to dwell on something as unsavoury as homosexuality results in its significance – which is often crucial to the understanding of individual texts – being missed. This perhaps partly explains what has happened in the cases of Marlowe and others cited above.

We are dealing, then, with critics who are reluctant to take gay issues seriously. It is therefore not surprising that the extraordinarily crucial question of homophobia amongst some feminist writers can be treated as of marginal interest. Thus, Patricia Craig, commenting on Bonnie Zimmerman's account of heterosexism in feminist writing, says: 'Is there no end to the prejudices needing to be rooted out of literary criticism?'[7] The implication is that anti-lesbian prejudice doesn't really 'count', isn't really as serious as, racism or sexism.

Embarrassment is often, of course, combined with ignorance. As late as 1977, Andrew Field treats us to quasi-medical opinions that ceased to be seriously held decades earlier. Writing about the family life of Vladimir Nabokov, he tells us that the author's father thought of homosexuality as an 'illness'; Field tells us that this is 'a view which is not universally accepted'. The father believed the 'illness' was transmitted by heredity and Field continues:

> It would appear now that V. D. Nabokov's attitude has much to be said for it, though in my mind I myself cannot disregard entirely the hothouse atmosphere in which the Nabokovs lived at the turn of the century and which seems to have allowed so many propensities of all manner and kind to grow and flourish exceptionally well. I hasten now (too slowly, thinks Nabokov) to leave this subject. The discomfiture which it caused decades ago in the Nabokov family has, at least in part, inspired an artistic interest in the subject which has provided a remarkable gallery of homosexual characters in Nabokov's writing.[8]

The horticultural metaphor is strong here; a 'hothouse atmosphere' is responsible for the determination of sexual choice. (In passing, we can note that the image is a favourite of those trying to get to grips with the prevalence of homosexual behaviour at single-sex boarding schools.) The word 'propensities' sounds as if it refers to something odd and faintly absurd, rather like the word 'tendencies'. Both words are still used by some people in referring to gay people; they are never used to describe heterosexual desire. The use of 'gallery' in the final sentence suggests in exactly what degree of esteem Field holds gay people.

Marginalisation sometimes seems to be the result of obtuseness rather than conscious prejudice. A startling recent case is Paul Zweig's recent and celebrated biography of Walt Whitman.[9] Zweig explains in his book that Whitman never seemed to like women and he quotes acquaintances who testify not only to this but to the fact that he seemed actually to dislike them. Zweig also explains that Whitman kept notebooks in which there are lists of details of scores of men, especially workers, soldiers and rough types, with short rapturous descriptions of their physical charms. He allows the overpowering and irrefutable evidence of the homoeroticism of the 'Calamus' poems. He concedes that Whitman loved men: 'Any love he experienced was for men, that's clear enough.'[10] Despite all this, Zweig talks of 'the Calamus poems and their *suggestion* [my italics] of homosexual love' and his conclusion is: 'Whitman's sexual life is still a mystery. Was he homosexual?'[11]

In many of the examples there is almost a kind of fear that the author under discussion must be saved from the 'taint' of homosexuality. Certainly the vociferousness and implausibility of these arguments needs some kind of explanation. Tom Marshall's comments on the following lines by D. H. Lawrence are a case in point. It is an early version of 'Cypresses', which appeared in *The Adelphi* for October 1923:

> Among the cypresses
> To sit with pure, slim, long-nosed,
> Evil-called, sensitive Etruscans, naked except for their boots;
> To be able to smile back at them
> And exchange the lost kiss
> And come to dark connection.[12]

To Marshall,

> This is open to obvious misunderstanding. Such a passage is probably best understood as the symbolic expression of an internal process by which Lawrence accepts and releases the qualities of his father which were driven underground in his youth.[13]

The 'misunderstanding' is Marshall's failure to take the poem for what it in fact is, an honest celebration of sexual desire. For such critics, writings descriptive of heterosexual love are *about* heterosexual love, whereas writings descriptive of homosexual love are metaphors for something completely different. Sexual desire is only seen as actually *counting* in a straight context.

This point also emerges in discussions of the 'Voyages' series of poems by Hart Crane, which were influenced by Crane's affair with Emil Opffer. The critic John Logan says: 'Crane is *not* writing simply of homosexual love or of one person.'[14] J. Unterecker says: 'Though the "Voyages" set is a consequence of a love for a man, its subject matter is love itself.'[15] S. Hazo gives quite a full account of why Crane's own experiences are irrelevant to our reading of the poems (reminiscent of introductions to school editions of Catullus and many another classical author, rejecting the homosexuality – by leaving it out – but glorying in the metre!):

> There is nothing in the poems that explicitly betrays a perversion of the impulses of love, and there is no thematic reason that would lead a reader to relate the love imagery, where it does exist, to a source homosexual in nature. Consequently, a reasonable reader could find no compelling factors in the six parts of 'Voyages' that would suggest that he consider the impulses of love in any but a heterosexual sense, regardless of the relationship that may have prompted them and regardless of the person to whom they may have been directed.[16]

Hazo is here claiming that *even though* it is not in contention that the genesis of the poem arose out of gay experience and desire, we are not as readers *forced* to read it as gay, and therefore we should read it as describing straight experience.

In addition to censorship and marginalisation, the homophobic critic will resort to raw abuse, expressed with a vehemence that is normally uncharacteristic of the writers I will cite. (For straights, homosexuality is always a *special case.* Remember Shelley, ready, even at the very real risk of imprisonment, to say and indeed publish almost anything, including vehement denunciation of the repulsive moral squalor, as he describes it, of Christianity; and yet he has a special rule for homosexuality. Remember also Jeremy Bentham, bravely publishing all manner of radical proposals in the same period, but stashing away thousands of pages of notes on homosexuality, so intimidated was he by the climate of opinion in Georgian England; a climate whose treatment of homosexuals makes the Victorians' public reaction to the Oscar Wilde trial appear benignly indulgent. For both men, the writing of even aloof academic essays was too intimidating.)[17]

Many reviews work on the abuse principle. The degree of vitriol they contain can still take us by surprise. The directness of the abuse is in contrast to the indirect, 'apologetic' and indeed often closeted nature of sexist and racist criticism. Take, for example, the reviewer Anthony Burgess. Speaking of a Paul Bowles biography, homosexuality is described as 'inversion'.[18] In a review of a Truman Capote biography, Capote's lover is a 'catamite', he himself is 'a little homosexual writer' and his feud with Gore Vidal is conducted 'in a vocabulary of homosexual abuse' (It is not explained what this might involve.)[19] The poet Roy Fuller, reviewing the *Penguin Book of Homosexual Verse,* calls an Auden poem 'limp-wristed'; other poets write works that come 'limping in'. He laments the very word 'gay' but accepts that, alas, it is 'seemingly now inevitable'. (This common obsession with the word 'gay' reflects a preference for the hate-laden alternatives; Fuller is sure that the word is 'not true' – that is, lesbian/gay people are miserable by nature.) He is happy with the erotic only if it is heterosexual; homoeroticism is 'ludicrous', 'obscene' and even 'pernicious'.[20] Professor Lord Quinton, writing about the memoirs of John Addington Symonds, finds the latter 'bent', his orientation being 'deplored proclivities'. Gay sex at Harrow is an 'iniquity'. He needs a 'cure'; his private life is 'weird', 'risible', but – wait for it – he deserves our 'sympathy'. A Latin don is 'queer'.[21] These are established writers writing in 'quality' newspapers. It is interesting to reflect that in the case of reviews concerning the interests of other minorities – black people, for example – sub-editors would soon snip out equivalent offensive words.

Abuse is not of course confined to reviews. In a full-length critical study, Iris Murdoch, whose novels are full of weird and neurotic gay characters, describes one of Sartre's gay characters as 'a pervert' who practises 'his vice', and, in this connection, complements the Frenchman on being 'a connoisseur of the abnormal'.[22] As late as 1983, the Proust translator Terence Kilmartin is describing de Charlus as an 'invert'.[23] George Steiner thinks of gay experience as 'the damned waste land of Sodom'.[24]

Feminist writers also offend. Betty Friedan, in one of the canonic texts of the new dispensation in sexual politics, *The Feminine Mystique,* mentions lesbians only once, and that in passing; the assumption is that homosexuality is essentially male. She tells us confidently: 'Male homosexuality was and is far more common than female homosexuality.'[25] She warns that homosexuality 'is spreading like a murky smog over the American scene'.[26]

Oppression sometimes relies on the tactic of making the victims appear as themselves delinquent or prejudiced. Thus, a favourite pre-emptive strike against gay men, forestalling our complaints of being the victims of discrimination, is to accuse us ourselves of discriminating against others. It is not surprising, then, that the old charge that gay men hate women occurs repeatedly in academic criticism. Discussing the poetry of Hart Crane, R. Lewis speaks of *The Wine Menagerie* in these terms: 'Such extreme male apprehension of female destructiveness was no doubt – in Crane's case – rooted in a homosexual element'[27] and again:

> Abstracting a human impulse from various of Crane's poems, one can easily enough explain the impulse, as in a case history, by reference to homosexuality; but this would rarely deepen one's understanding of the poem itself. Such a method would yield particularly obvious results with 'The Wine Menagerie' – a real-life sense of woman as lethal, as wanting in fact to cut one's head off, is patently homosexual in origin. But this is not what the *poem* is about.[28]

Here we have, firstly, the myth of the gay man's fear and

loathing of women; secondly, the medicalising of sexuality through phrases such as 'as in a case history'; thirdly, sexual orientation is not really important for Lewis because he wants to enjoy the poem but cannot really do so because his attitude towards homosexuality gets in the way. His answer – the one scholars have been employing for decades – is to say that the gender of the loved one is of no consequence, that the work has a universal meaning and appeal, by which is always meant a heterosexual meaning and appeal. The truth of this hypothesis can be tested quite simply by asking oneself whether in a work dealing with heterosexual experience (*Romeo and Juliet* for example), the gender of the loved one is considered of no consequence in determining its effect or its meaning.

A favourite abuse strategy is derogatory juxtaposition. Almost every study of Hart Crane speaks of his alcoholism and his sexuality in the same breath: 'he was an alcoholic and a homosexual' (A. Alvarez); 'Even towards the end, he never completely gave up the struggle against his two weaknesses, alcohol and homosexuality' (Susan Jenkins Brown); 'as his drinking became more furious, so did his homosexual liaisons, chiefly with sailors, become more squalid, more dangerous, and more hopeless' (R. W. Butterfield); 'uneducated, alcoholic, homosexual, paranoic, suicidal' (L. S. Dembo); 'Sexual aberration and drunkenness were the pitfalls in which his spirit wrestled with a kind of desperation' (W. Fowlie); 'This vice, together with his alcoholism . . . tended not only to weaken but to age him'; 'His homosexuality grew intense and his bouts of drunkenness multiplied'; 'His final leap from the "Orizaba" exceeded his homosexuality and his alcoholism not so much in intent as in degree'; 'The poet could . . . descend for days into drunkenness and perversion' (S. Hazo); 'his addiction to homosexuality and alcohol' (V. Quinn); 'his exhibitionistic homosexuality, his alcoholism, his hysterical relations with friends and lovers and family, and finally his suicide at the age of thirty-three' (M. L. Rosenthal – this last even makes the *age* of the suicide seem like a glance at the sort of behaviour that can be expected from a gay man); 'The increasing disorder of his personal life, dominated by alcoholism and homosexuality' (M. K. Spears); 'He was certainly homosexual, however, and he became a chronic and extreme alcoholic. I should judge that he cultivated these weaknesses on principle' (Yvor Winters).[29]

Writing about Proust, Valerie Minogue speaks of 'the snobbery of Legrandin, the cruelty of Françoise, the lesbianism of Mlle Vinteuill'.[30] She speaks of two Prousts; there is Proust 'the asthmatic' and also Proust 'the homosexual and neurotic'.[31] A recent review of a book on Thomas Mann tells us: 'He was homosexual. He was a drug addict.'[32]

Even where critics seem to intend no offence, the assumptions underlying what they write make their position clear. For example, the biographer of T. E. Lawrence tells us: 'We had devoted one chapter to the *charge* [my italics][33] that Lawrence was a homosexual.' Eugenia Collier, attacking what she sees as the coarseness of James Baldwin's novel *Another Country,* says that there is 'something offensive for everyone . . . be it the sordidly graphic descriptions of sex, the detailed treatment of homosexuality or the degrading references to race'.[34] Sex (presumably heterosexual, another interesting assumption) is offensive if it is sordid or graphically described; references to race are offensive if they are degrading; but homosexuality is just offensive *per se.* In a review of the novel *Killing Orders* by Sara Paretsky, Christopher Wordsworth tells us about 'the murder of a good lesbian friend (relax, our girl is 'straight' as a die)'.[35] The parentheses here are based on the assumption that the potential readers of this novel – all of whom are presumed to be heterosexual – would be ill at ease or simply unprepared to accept a lesbian as a central character. (Incidentally, 'our girl' is itself full of patriarchal resonances.)

I should like to conclude this chapter with an extended examination of a particular case, the critic Jeffrey Meyers, whose writings illustrate many of the points that I have made above. Meyers has published a full-length study of homosexuality in literature. This is from the opening of that study:

> I have no desire to praise or condemn homosexuality; and do not imply a moral judgement when I use words like invert, pederast and perverse, which have negative connotations. I do hope, however, to maintain the sympathetic attitude that is necessary to understand any work of art.[36]

From the very start the writer hereby asserts his own heterosexuality, reminiscent of the way actors playing lesbian or gay roles insist on giving interviews and mentioning as if casually that, of course, they themselves are not homosexual. The effect in both cases is to suggest that, while these people might have a professional or cultural connection with homosexuality, they would not want it to be thought to touch them more closely. Whether it is done consciously or not, the idea clearly emerges of the gay experience as tainted.

Secondly, Meyers renders homosexuality problematic; it would make no sense in our culture to say, 'I have no desire to praise or condemn heterosexuality', because the issue of potential condemnation never arises. Meyers here actually announces his negative view of homosexuality in the very phrase that purports to be disinterested.

Thirdly, he tries to excuse himself for using the terms of grossest abuse. However, it is not at all clear what possible reason he has for actually using them other than to employ them in their natural function: that of gross abuse. Even popular Fleet Street newspapers had, by the 1970s, abandoned 'inverts' as a term, and 'pederast' is especially malign for a specific reason of its own. This is that the word has two senses: in one it refers to the lovers of young boys (often of an age that renders sexual experiences with them liable to criminal prosecution in many countries) but it is also used simply to mean 'male homosexual'. It is of course a classic device of spurious reasoning to use a word ostensibly employing one of its meanings (usually the one deemed less offensive) while actually evoking the other. The speaker evades liability because the ambiguity of the word is an escape clause; but the damage has been done. In any case, other writings by Meyers show that he is happy to use the word 'fairy' unironically and out of quotation marks to refer to gay men.[37] (And we note that critics who have cold feet over the use of racist terminology – 'nigger' and so on – do not hesitate with the homophobic equivalents. I do not here necessarily mean Mr Meyers, who may have very benign views on racial questions.) The last sentence of the quoted extract carries the clear implication that the 'sympathetic attitude' is against the grain, a difficult task requiring some stomach: he has to force himself to it. 'Sympathetic' itself is of course a code-word; it is often found side by side with another favourite word – 'compassionate' – applied by straight critics to films and novels that condescend to the gay experience.

Further evidence of the same approach emerges in a later

piece, Meyers's review of Gregory Woods's *Articulate Flesh,*[38] which is a study of gay literature. His general approach is that homosexual writers have been interesting in the past because the tortured guilt and pain that is the natural corollary of their pitiful state gives rise to angst-filled literature of the first quality. However, more modern writers, emerging from a Western culture in which the beginnings of an acceptance of the idea of equality irrespective of sexual orientation is evident, have switched in their writings from expressing guilt and self-loathing to celebrating their sexual identity and moving more vigorously onto the attack against the anti-libertarian lobbies. This 'pride' is denounced by Meyers. Thus, he attacks Woods for recom mending to us the later poems of Thom Gunn. We are told that these sexually explicit poems are 'not nearly as good as his early work, written when he was in the closet'.[39] He goes on to quote sexually explicit passages from an assortment of poets, also quoted by Woods, as if his mere requoting of them before an audience (the readers of the *Journal of English and Germanic Philology*) which – and this is surely another equally telling indicator of the state of academic sentiment towards the gay minority – is assumed to share his hostility, will be sufficient to establish their absurdity and tastelessness. The extent of his prudery can be gauged from the fact that he describes the swallowing of semen as part of the 'squalid side' of gay sex.[40]

Meyers takes an extended interest in matters only tangentially connected with the contents of the book. Meyers himself could not deny that in his review he has deliberately attempted to couple his criticisms of the contents with his criticisms of these other matters in order to render his attack all the stronger. Thus, he complains that the book has been published without proper publishers' permissions and acknowledgements. He tells us that the dust-wrapper is inappropriate, amongst other things, because the two men pictured on the front of it are not 'sensual fleshy men' and they are 'fully clothed'.[41] One can only guess at his meaning here – perhaps it is a received thing with him that gay men are never slim and rarely wear clothes – except that it seems he is adducing entirely non-academic criteria (such as the design of a dust-jacket, over which, notoriously, authors have little control) to damn an academic study.

Meyers also tells us that Woods 'does not seem to realise that it was and is potentially libellous to mention the homosexuality of a living writer, particularly one who has not publicly acknowledged it'.[42] Again, this cannot provide unambiguous evidence of any such views on Meyers's own part, but he does seem to lay himself open to the danger of it being thought that he himself regards the mere fact of someone's being gay as a blot on their character. If this were indeed the case, then the whole edifice on which his work is based might be seen to be flawed. Meyers concludes his review thus:

> Hart Crane's honest description of desperate fumblings for relief in dark, public places and his degrading image of homosexual love as a matchstick spinning in the piss of a urinal, as well as the young Auden's sad confession of the deliberately superficial, venal, and exploititive aspects of one-night stands . . . are more moving and meaningful than the entire volume of Woods's cant. Moreover, the reader of Woods's book is ineluctably influenced by a word he never mentions, AIDS, which can be contracted by seminal ingestion and anal penetration, and has reinforced, among many homosexuals, centuries of fear, revulsion and guilt.[43]

The reference to AIDS that closes the review is quite extraordinary, for it is no part of the stated aims of the study under review to deal with the impact of AIDS. It is as if one were reviewing a book on the medieval religious ceremonies of Caribbean islanders, and threw in for good measure the fact that some of the islanders' descendants were engaged in street robberies in London in the 1990s, designed to generate hostile sentiment. In the use of the words 'fear, revulsion and guilt', Meyers manages to make it sound as if these emotions are the natural and inevitable consequences of a gay lifestyle – it is for this reason that he links them directly with sexual activity – whereas, in so far as they do exist in gay men, they are the result of direct oppression from church, state, the establishment and society generally. Meyers speaks of the existence of gay men who feel 'fear, revulsion and guilt' in such a way as to raise the suspicion that for him, these are the correct and 'natural' emotions for homosexual men, and that personal sexual liberation doctrines are anathema.[44] A key phrase in the review is, of course, the 'degrading image of homosexual love as a matchstick spinning in the piss of a urinal', which is effectively

Meyers's image of it. Anything celebrating the sexual aspect of homosexuality is therefore, for Meyers, repellant. The following passage from his own book explains satisfactorily why the earlier works were favoured:

> The naturalistic and documentary descriptions in the works of contemporary writers like Jean Genet and William Burroughs, John Rechy and Hubert Selby, are very different from the novels discussed in this book. They concern the homosexual's acts and *not his mind,* and appeal to sensation rather than imagination. [They] deliberately abandon the very qualities of subtlety, ambiguity and restraint that distinguish the artistic greatness of the earlier works. When the laws of obscenity were changed and homosexuality became legal, apologies seemed inappropriate, the theme surfaced defiantly and sexual acts were grossly described. The emancipation of the homosexual has led, paradoxically, to the decline of his art.[45]

Meyers's work is representative of an entire school of criticism that gives approval to literary texts which duplicate mainstream moral values, and to withhold that approval from those which challenge or disrupt those values. In this light, it is clear why the earlier gay books are so much more satisfactory. Instead of erotic celebration there is fear and disgust, instead of openness there is closetry, instead of assertiveness and joy there is negativity and pain.

The strength of these deeply imbued views can hardly be exaggerated; they can, unfortunately, always be demonstrated. Oliver Bernard tells us: 'I do not think that his [the poet Rimbaud's] homosexuality matters nearly as much as what sort of person he was.'[46]

Academic and lower-level journalistic criticism has predictably taken its cue from the wider culture. It is therefore especially important to develop the field of gay studies, so that critical perspectives based on positive values, tolerance and a pleasure in human diversity can balance the damaging effect of the majority of studies currently available.

2

The Legacy of Byron and Wilde

George Gordon (Lord) Byron (1788–1824) was brought up by his mother, his father having deserted the family during his childhood. At the age of ten, he inherited the barony, and moved from very modest accommodation to the semi-ruined abbey which was the family seat. He went to Harrow and Cambridge, and during these early years experienced loving attachments to fellow pupils and students. An unrequited love for a young woman in his youth left a permanent bitterness. His first privately printed collection of poems (Hours of Idleness) *was badly received in 1807, but on the publication of the first two cantos of* Childe Harold *(1812) he became famous almost overnight. His incestuous relationship with his half-sister Augusta, and the dismal failure of his marriage to the rich Annabella Milbanke, led to scandal and, combined with his disgust at English society's hypocrisy, this led to his departure from England. He finally settled in Italy, where he had many heterosexual love affairs, the most durable with Teresa, Countess Guiccioli. During his life, especially abroad, he also had several less well-documented homosexual relationships and passions – not always reciprocated – and this aspect of his life is reflected in some of his poetry, as we shall see below. He supported Italian revolutionaries, and played a key role in the Greek struggle against the Turks until his death of fever in 1824.*

Oscar Wilde (1854–1900) was born in Dublin and educated at Oxford, where he was under the spell of Walter Pater and aestheticism. He published a collection of poems in 1881 and later in the same decade a number of short stories. His first major work, The Picture of Dorian Gray *(1891), caused a scandal because of its general 'decadence' and, more specifically, its blatancy about homosexuality. He became successful with a series of social comedies such as* The Ideal Husband *(1895) and* The Importance of Being Earnest *(1895). Also in 1895, after two famous trials, he was sentenced to two years' imprisonment for homosexual 'offences', as a result of which he wrote 'The Ballad of Reading Gaol' (1898) and 'De Profundis' (1905). He died in Paris in 1900.*

BYRON

> *And mortals dared to ponder for themselves . . . and to speak*
> *Of freedom, the forbidden fruit*
>
> (Byron, *Manfred*)

Running as a persistent theme through the literary works which will be examined in this book, is the notion of human freedom as forbidden. The extract from Byron's verse drama, *Manfred,* quoted above, clearly evokes the fall of Adam and Eve after their eating the forbidden apple. For Byron, as for the writer of Genesis, the pursuit of freedom exacts an awful price; one which only the most reckless are prepared to pay. How far this daring is present in the literary characters studied in this book, and how far the theme of daring itself can be associated with a gay sensibility present in the writers of these works, are questions which readers should keep in the forefront of their minds. As I proceed in this study, I shall make connections forwards and backwards between the writers under discussion, hoping to consolidate and emphasise such similarities as exist in this regard.

Although this book concerns the writers of this century, it is useful to begin with certain observations on Byron and Wilde. Byron created, in a series of works, a particular type, the defiant Romantic hero, thus establishing a pattern both of attitude and behaviour which is closely reflected in most of the gay works of the twentieth century which are the subject of this book. Byron was bisexual; most of his sexual experiences were with women, and those with men all probably occurred abroad. Some of my remarks below have been inspired by a very fine study of Byron's life and work from the gay perspective.[1] It is not surprising that Byron's heterosexual experience should be constantly adduced by critics in order to shed light on his poetry, whilst his gay experiences are seen as marginal and, sometimes, uncharacteristic. The effect of this critical tradition is to miss important aspects of Byron's work, as I try to show below.

I have divided my comments on Byron into two sections. In the first, I give a general descriptive account of the characteristics of a typical Byronic hero, based on the narrative poem *The Corsair* and its hero Conrad. These characteristics, and the issues raised by them, recur in the texts discussed in the remaining chapters of this book. In the second section, I offer a gay reading of the narrative poem *Lara*

From the beginning of *The Corsair* Conrad's reckless physical courage is presented, mixed with an entirely unapologetic malice against an enemy: 'No dread of death if with us die our foes' (1, l. 23). This is combined with an asceticism which is seen as nourishing the mind:

> Earth's coarsest bread, the garden's homeliest roots,
> And scarce the summer luxury of fruits,
> His short repast in humbleness supply
> With all a hermit's board would scarce deny.
> But while he shuns the grosser joys of sense,
> His mind seems nourish'd by that abstinence . . .
> (1, ll. 71–6)

Akin to this is Lara's disdain for 'shadowy honour', 'substantial gain', 'beauty's preference' and a 'rival's pain'. This disposition is not unconnected with a further trait, pride, for the disregard of those things for which the generality of mankind longs, shows a kind of arrogant self-assuredness. This pride is especially well set out in stanza eight. There we find a theory of human hierarchy very similar to that espoused by D. H. Lawrence in his later years. Certain people are born to govern, others to serve. Those who serve should be content (they usually are in Byron) to be led by the strong captain, even to death: 'And who dare question aught that he decides?' (1, l. 172). The pride of this leader puts an enormous distance between him and his followers:

> Still sways their souls with that commanding art
> That dazzles, leads, yet chills the vulgar heart.
> (1, ll. 177–8)

It is in the fitness of things, a kind of natural law, that 'The many still must labour for the one' (1, l. 188). The strange mechanism by which the leader exerts his power over potentially rebellious followers is found in 'The power of Thought – the magic of the mind' (1, l. 182). The relationship between the leader and the led is less that of voluntary accord, more that of an inevitable state of affairs based on relative strength. Conrad 'moulds another's weakness to [his] will' (1, l. 184). The stanza ends with an insistence that the leader be not 'accused' by virtue of wielding this power in the manner described:

> 'Oh! if he [the follower] knew the weight of splendid chains,
> How light the balance of his humbler pains!.
>
> (1, ll. 191–2)

For Byron's narrator, this pride is justified; one can see it (*pace* Shakespeare) in the face and carriage. Those who 'paused to look again' (1, l. 199) at their leader could see 'more than marks the crowd of vulgar men' (1, l. 200). The view advanced here of the relationship between leader and led is consistent with what in our own century is identified as fascism.

The leader retains his power and respect by standing haughtily aloof; he is 'That man of loneliness and mystery' (1, l. 173). The mystery is important, for Byron stresses the ineffable; a point to which, in his work, he repeatedly returns. Conrad's features

> perplex'd the view,
> As if within that murkiness of mind
> Work'd feelings fearful, and yet undefined.
>
> (1, ll. 210–12)

The notion of the ineffable is perhaps linked to the next characteristic. The piracy of Conrad, and the crimes it entails, leads to guilt. Byron's work in general is ambiguous here, because, mirroring exactly his attitude to the events of his own life, he combines an existentialist's disregard for the moral norms of society, and a determination to follow his inner impulses wherever they may lead (usually they lead into evil and criminality), with an experience of guilt for the resulting behaviour. This seems paradoxical (surely guilt presumes acceptance of society's norms?) until we realise two things (both of them also potent in the works of both Wilde and Genet): the first is that certain courses of action are deliberately chosen precisely because they produce that sense of guilt which, by its very power, reinforces in the doer the exhilarating experience of having chosen freely in the teeth of society's dicta. The second is that guilt, frequently described as though it were one thing, is in fact two. There is the intellectual recognition of wrongdoing and the consequent emotional regret or remorse; and then there is that state of mind suffered by victims (victims of rape, for example, or the gay and Jewish survivors of the extermination camps in the Second World War) who frequently attest to feelings of 'guilt'. It is this second sense of guilt, almost universal amongst gay people reared in a homophobic tradition, which informs the work of Byron and those writers (like Wilde and Genet) who come after him.

It is of related interest to note here how in Byron's life there is a tension; he desires both conformity and freedom. During his time in Venice, he was simultaneously acting the public role of the adulterer, whilst insisting that his daughter be strictly reared by nuns in a Catholic convent.

Guilt and aloof behaviour in the Byronic hero combine to produce another characteristic, which is the desire to conceal: 'Still seems there something he would not have seen' (1, l. 208); and later, 'Too close inquiry his stern glance would quell' (1, l. 214). Conrad's desire to conceal is matched by that of Byron's narrator, and Byron himself, who withhold the tantalising secrets of Conrad from the readers of the poem. This is another noticeably paradoxical area for Byron, for, as we shall see in the case of *Lara*, the desire to conceal is matched by an equally strong desire to disclose.

A contempt for society, and a general misanthropy, also characterise Conrad: 'He hated man too much to feel remorse' (1, l. 262). Indeed, he goes as far as saying that the possibility of sustaining his love for Medora is actually based on his hatred of everyone else: 'I cease to love thee when I love mankind' (1, l. 405). To act dramatically, preferably in physical danger and for no merely materialistic reward – this is the goal. (It is useful here to compare Conrad with another Byronic pirate, the Selim of 'The Bride of Abydos', who has taken to piracy not from greed, but because amongst the outlaws is to be found 'open speech, and ready hand,/Obedience to their chief's command',

'Friendship', 'faith to all', vengeance exacted against those who kill members of the band, and, amongst those who are 'Distinguish'd from the vulgar ranks' certain 'higher thoughts' and 'visionary schemes' are forthcoming.)

Conrad (perhaps Byron, endlessly echoing Shakespearean diction and themes, is thinking of the Conrad of *Much Ado About Nothing*) is an embittered melancholic. The result is an intense malice:

> [Conrad] thought the voice of wrath a sacred call,
> To pay the injuries of some on all
>
> (1, ll. 263–4)

Or, as we hear earlier, 'There was a laughing Devil in his sneer' (1, l. 223). During the attack on his arch-enemy Seyd, Conrad asks: 'Their galleys blaze – why not their city too?' (11, l. 195). His slaughter of the Muslims is done with relish. A troubled conscience is seen as a liability. We are told, memorably, 'the weak alone repent!' (11, l. 335). Yet, despite all this, Byron wants to balance this dark picture of Conrad by two further characteristics: his utter faithfulness in his love for Medora, and the insistence that Conrad is 'naturally' good, but has been 'Warp'd by the world in Disappointment's school' (1, l. 253)

Anyone who has read a life of Byron will recognise most of these characteristics of Conrad as, *mutatis mutandis*, shared by the author. This is of course not to say that Byron is necessarily consciously aware of this, although I believe he is. Byron's exciting, extremely various, sexually adventurous and scandalous life is metaphorically rendered through the piratical life of Conrad. These characteristics of the Byronic hero inform the spirit of subsequent literature to an extraordinary extent. The bitter misanthropy and the criminality in Genet spring from this tradition. So does the determined commitment of Tennessee Williams to show his audiences that moral conventions and cultural norms can be hideously constricting; so does Wilde's Dorian Gray, in his pursuit of evil as a kind of defiant self-indulgence linked with a Faustian pride, and eagerness for discovery. We see Conrad again in Orton's contempt for sexual propriety and hard work, in Cavafy's delicious promiscuity, in Baldwin's *J'accuse* hurled against the hypocrisy of his fellow Americans. Even in the milder strains – the gentle pleas for tolerance from Forster, Isherwood and Leavitt – we hear echoes of Conrad's disdain for both the masses and the rulers, in their collaboration to fix and enforce limitations to the human spirit.

Crompton's book on Byron, cited above, gives comprehensive treatment to the way in which the poet's sexual desire for men is expressed in the writings. Here, I should like to examine one of the narrative poems to show how this approach might work in detail. The most promising and suggestive, *Lara* (1812), was published after Byron's grand tour of Portugal, Spain, Greece, and Turkey, between 1809 and 1811. The eponymous hero shares many of Conrad's characteristics: surly and aloof, a past life shrouded in mystery, a disdain for the society of others, a natural quality of leadership inspiring others to give him total loyalty, blood-thirstiness, being 'naturally' good until corrupted by the world, someone who has drunk deep of the cup of life, and someone, above all, with a guilty secret.

Lara also shares with Conrad a desire for death. The latter, for example, prefers to contemplate a painful end preceded by torture rather than vanquish his foe in a way which seems to him underhand. When captured:

> His sole regret the life he still possest;
> His wounds too slight, though taken with that will,
> Which would have kiss'd the hand that then could kill.
> (11, ll. 287–9)

A little earlier in the poem, we have read of the 'happier dead' (11, l. 274). Lara, too, after plunging into youthful excesses (typically, unspecified), 'awoke' from this frenzied period of indulgence 'To curse the wither'd heart that would not break' (1, l. 130). The pursuit of sensation, according to *Lara,* is an attempt by the individual to subject himsef to emotional and physical extremes which will hopefully blot out the experience of perceiving the world as meaningless – a perception which has set in during youth, and which can be traced back to Byron's own highly disturbed childhood and adolescence (abandoned by his father; seduced by his nurse at the age of nine; highly sensitive about his lame foot; fraught relationship with his mother). Both Wilde and Genet offer in their writings clear later examples of characters, in some measure reflecting the dispositions of their creators, who act in this sort of way, defensively, against the meaninglessness of the world.

The eponymous hero of the poetic drama *Manfred* (1817) has a craving for death even stronger than Lara's. When one of the seven spirits offers Manfred 'Kingdom and sway, and strength, and length of days' he is interrupted impatiently: 'Accursed! what have I to do with days?/They are too long already' (1, i, 167–169). He later says it is 'my fatality to live' (1, ii, 24), and when the Abbot in Act 11 says 'Thy life's in peril', he has a simple answer: 'Take it' (111, i, 46–7).

It is in this resentful spirit, of having to continue a life without apparent purpose, that Lara returns to his kingdom from a mysterious sojourn in an unspecified foreign land. He is accompanied by a fanatically devoted servant from this foreign country, called Khaled. (The name entitles us, especially in view of the Oriental seting of several Byron tales, to assume that the unspecified country is an Islamic one. This is important, for Byron clearly recognised Islamic societies as lacking in the sexual hysteria of the West.) Isolated and disdainful as he is, only Khaled really seems to understand Lara. There is repeated emphasis on their special bond, and the fact that occasionally they talk in the foreign language which none but they can understand.

The plot of the tale is complex but its main thrust is that, having returned to the kingdom after many years away (having led a life of debauchery and indulgence in the unspecified foreign country), Lara's tranquility is shattered by the arrival at a festival (which he attends reluctantly, maintaining the aloof disdain of the Byronic hero) of a man, Ezzelin, who is on the verge of denouncing him publicly for some hideous deed which the reader presumes has been committed by Lara in the foreign country. Ezzelin is murdered before he can fulfil his threat, and the narrator hints that Lara is responsible. Ezzelin's ally Otho then orchestrates a rebellion against Lara during which the latter is mortally wounded. He dies in Khaled's arms. Khaled subsequently dies of grief at his master's death.

I want to give a reading of *Lara* informed largely by the biographical approach. Lara's experiences and attitudes, both on the simple factual level, but also on the psychological level, provide an accurate key to understanding Byron and his work.

Byron's incestous relationship with his half-sister Augusta, and his homosexual desires and acts, created in him that sense of exhilerating freedom, combined with overpowering guilt, which I have described as a part of the character of the typical Byronic hero. The other characteristics – haughtiness, preference for solitude, habits of secrecy, misanthropy and so on – can easily be seen to fit the disposition of someone consciously acting against some of the most sacred moral principles of his society. Even more than Conrad, Lara is a startling self-portrait in many ways.

Lara guards a terrible, unrevealed secret (he appears to be prepared to kill – if indeed he is responsible for Ezzelin's death – to protect it), just as Byron did where his sex life was concerned. Ezzelin represents in the poem Byron's fear of discovery. It is not surprising that for Lara: 'Not much he loved long question of the past,/Nor told of wondrous wilds, and deserts vast . . .' (1, ll. 85–6). The close verbal echo of Shakespeare's Othello here – see the speech at 1, iii, 128ff. – is appropriate, for the black Venetian general represents in so many respects a man who is an integral part of the society and indeed of its establishment, and yet in other ways so hopelessly an outsider. This isolation means that

> He did not follow what they all pursued
> With hope still baffled, still to be renew'd;
> Nor shadowy honour, nor substantial gain,
> Nor beauty's preference, and the rival's pain:
> Around him some mysterious circle thrown
> Repell'd approach, and showed him still alone;
> Upon his eye sat something of reproof,
> That kept at least frivolity aloof . . .
>
> (1, ll. 102–10)

Lara's contempt for the vulgar masses – 'The men with whom he felt condemned to breath' (1, l. 346) – is also a celebrated feature of the poet. Despite his oft-touted radicalism in Parliament, Byron was insufferably snobbish. He once referred contemptuously to the writer and lawyer Francis Jeffrey as having been 'born in a garret sixteen stories high'.[2]

Lara and Byron were both deserted by their fathers in childhood; both were, in a sense, exiles. Both throw themselves vigorously into life. Lara was 'Burning for pleasure, not averse from strife' (1, l. 116), and from these extremes of conduct 'he did awake/To curse the wither'd heart that would not break' (1, ll. 129–30). This final line conjures up the youthful Byron suffering terribly from that unrequited love for a woman which embittered him to the end of his days.

I make this identification between Lara and the poet not only because the characteristics of the Byronic hero thus become autobiographical, but because if we accept the close link, we can see Lara's relationship with Khaled as expressing many of Byron's own thoughts and feelings about same-sex love.

Khaled is alien. He shares the strange language with his master and no one else. He is from an Islamic culture which, given Byron's experience in Turkey of the Muslim attitude to homosexuality, is especially significant. It can serve two purposes at once: to represent in a kind of code, perhaps only for himself, or for those few of his friends for whom the Orient evoked homosexuality (his letters, extremely carefully worded for fear of official interception of the post, speak of this frequently), the idea of a secret lover. The second purpose is to give an ethnic explanation of Khaled's total love and devotion to his master, as homophobic readers might suspect such devotion between two Europeans. These two purposes are, typically for Byron, contradictory. Specifically, as mentioned above, they represent the poet's desire both to reveal and to conceal his thoughts on sexuality.

The Oriental character is a contrast to the European, who is jaded, vulgar, boring, heart-breaking and with whom love is impossible. Khaled represents fidelity, simplicity, intensity of feeling, courage, pure love: the attributes Byron despaired of finding in England. Particularly important is Khaled's sharing the secret guiltiness of Lara, or at least what is called a 'secret care' (1, l. 534). Stanza xxvii, Canto 1, shows us Khaled as a kind of mirror-image of his master. It is true that he is in the role of servant, but he does this from devotion rather than from mercenary considerations. He is sensitive, guessing Lara's needs before they are spoken; and he shares Lara's disdain for 'the menial train' (1, l. 568). Daringly (because the relationship between the two men must hereby be more likely to be inferred as sexual as a result) the poem dwells on Khaled's physical beauty. He has a delicate shape, blushing cheeks which are tanned but not excessively, sparkling eyes and long eyelashes. More suggestively still, 'For hours on Lara he would fix his gaze' (1, l. 544).

Thus, we can say that Byron is using the idea of the Orient, as embodied in the character of Khaled, as a metaphor for the possibility of gay love, but because the poem is being published in a country where such a possibility is unthinkable, this theme cannot be presented except indirectly. Part of the indirectness is a kind of misleading of the reader, because the 'Oriental' virtues of fidelity, courage and so on, are virtues associated with certain cultures (ancient Greece, the Samurai tradition of Japan) which have a quasi-respectable cult of warriors loving youths 'purely'. There is a tradition of gay writers (for example, T. E. Lawrence and A. E. Houseman) evoking male comradeship in this way as a means of suggesting the homoerotic without getting into censorship problems.

The whole issue becomes much more complex in *Lara* because, at the end of the poem, when Khaled faints after Lara dies in his arms, it is discovered that Khaled is really a woman. (Retrospectively, we remember the ambiguous clues to this, such as Khaled's hand being described as 'So femininely white it might bespeak/Another sex . . .' (1, ll. 576–7).) This revelation might seem to render my reading of the meaning of the poem absurd. Khaled, it is usually argued, is to be compared to the Gulnare of *The Corsair*, an oriental woman whose devotion is so intense that it can survive on total service to the loved one without any possibilty of reciprocation. (Conrad already loves another, Medora.) However, my view is that Byron wants his readers, during the actual process of reading the poem, to feel (of course with different degrees of awareness) the homoerotic force of the relationship between characters both of whom they are sure are men. Retrospectively, of course, once the revelation of Khaled's identity has been made, this view must be revised – but Byron has ensured that the readers have already had the experience (exhilarating to some, shocking to others) of assuming a love between two men. It is quite possible that Byron's making Khaled a woman, and revealing this at the end, is a kind of funk. He knows what the poem is really about, but can't risk so obvious a revelation of the nature of his own desires. In Byron's *The Bride of Abydos* – which hints at incest between Selim and his sister Zuleika – we see something of the same process, dictated by Byron's desire to speak about his own feelings for his half-sister, but not too directly.

I should like to conclude with a few comments on *The Episode of Nisus and Euryalus,* Byron's loose translation of a passage in Book IX of Vergil's *Aeneid,* dealing with a heroic martial exploit involving valour, loyalty and love between the two men of the title. Comparing the original with Byron's version, we can see occasional changes of emphasis which bear out the covert way in which the poet articulates a gay sensibility.

We can readily see what attracted Byron about this passage in Vergil: the youth and beauty of the two warriors, their utter devotion and courage, the idea of fighting in order to maintain and consolidate the love and esteem between friends. In Vergil, Nisus is largely motivated in his desire to go on the dangerous mission by a desire for material rewards. Byron plays this down dramatically. Similarly, Euryalus' desire for glory ('smit with a mighty love of glory' in Vergil) is changed entirely ('With equal ardour fired', l. 37). When Iulus, a chieftain, is promising Nisus male slaves to toil for him, and twelve women captives for his sexual pleasure, Byron's wording suggests that both men and women will provide the sex:

> twelve slaves, and twice six captive dames,
> To soothe thy softer hours with amorous flames.
> (ll. 159–60)

Towards the end, when Nisus sees that Euryalus is in danger, he feels a desire to die with him in battle – and Byron adds, what is not in Vergil, 'for whom he wish'd to live' (l. 338). Nisus does indeed throw himself into certain death by confronting a numerous band of the enemy, enraged that they have killed his friend. Mortally wounded, he throws himself on his friend's body. Vergil has: 'he threw himself on his lifeless friend . . . and there at last reposed in tranquil death'. Byron gives us [my italics]:

> Thus Nisus all his fond affection proved –
> Dying revenged the fate of him he loved;
> Then on his bosom sought his *wonted* place,
> And death was heavenly in his friend's embrace!

It is commonplace for literary works (to say nothing of the language of 'democratic' politics, and indeed ordinary social discourse) to provide a hidden subtext quite at variance with the 'official' meaning, which is provided as a cover of safety out of fear of censorship or fear of self-revelation. Marlowe's *Doctor Faustus* is an example: officially it views the eponymous hero as evil and damned; but the feeling of the work is in favour of Faustus' atheistic defiance. Milton's depiction of Satan in *Paradise Lost* is often thought to be another example. Sartre's play *Les Mouches,* written in France during the German occupation in the Second World War, actually attacks fascism whilst pretending to be a mere reworking of the Orestes story. Recognising the overwhelming desire to speak of what is so central to his emotional life, combined with a caution and fear which casts ambiguity over the subject matter, is an important key to understanding much of Byron's poetry.

WILDE

Wilde accepts the basic premise on which Byron's tales are based: that English society is stultifying and freedom and fulfilment can only come through disdain and defiance of it. But whereas Byron's tales take place outside English society (his heroes are pirates and rebels in foreign lands) Wilde presents in *The Picture of Dorian Gray*[3] a story of the subverting of that society from within. Another point of comparison is that Wilde felt able to be much more direct than Byron in suggesting that outlawed sexual desire is the root cause from which proceeds a much wider condemnation of society's norms. In effect, this greater directness means that nobody reading the novel at the time of its publication (unless they affected disingenuousness) was in any doubt about the homosexual desires of the three central male characters (Basil Hallward, Lord Henry Wotton and Dorian himself) or about the sexual 'crimes' which Dorian indulges in. However, Wilde stops short of making absolutely explicit the sexual aspect of homosexuality – a necessary precaution. His extraordinary risk in publishing such a novel was balanced by a fear of his sexual orientation being discovered. This contradiction – a powerful instinct to tell the truth, and another powerful instinct of self-preservation against the mob – is precisely what we have seen in Byron's tales.

Although homophobia was less fanatical in Wilde's time than in Byron's,[4] it was still demented and terrible. The writer Beverley Nichols, who was a boy not long after the publication of *Dorian Gray*, was once discovered by his father reading the novel:

> In an ecstasy of incoherent rage, his father proceeded to spit repeatedly on the pages until his chin was covered with saliva; then he lifted the book to his mouth, and dismembered it with his teeth. When his innocent son bravely persisted in demanding what it was that Oscar Wilde had done, he received the answer written on a scrap of paper: *Illum crimen horribile . . . quod non nominandum est.* [This horrible crime . . . which is not to be named.][5]

Quod non nominandum est. This phrase, used for centuries in English secular and ecclesiastical law, is behind the later expression ('the love that dare not speak its name') of Lord Alfred Douglas. The idea of speaking the unspeakable lies behind many of the energies of gay writing.

Dorian Gray is a novel with many literary sources; so many that, combined with its complex melodramatic plot and (often seriously irritating) epigrams, it is difficult to get a sense of the work's coherence. The central allegory, of the painting of Dorian Gray which will grow old instead of the man himself, has been the subject of many varied interpretations. It certainly has at least some elements of a Faustian, un-Godly pact with the forces of evil. Indeed, Marlowe's play of *Doctor Faustus* is relevant here in another way. To placate the official culture, Marlowe, as we saw above, has to describe Faustus's defiance as wicked, but the subtext seems to celebrate his actions. Wilde, too, uses the vocabulary of the official culture much of the time, so that Dorian Gray 'ruins' men, is 'depraved', launches into 'evil', and so on. But we would be foolish to take this at face value.

Critics protective of heterosexist culture do, however, take it at face value. For Jeffrey Meyers, the novel is about 'the impossibility of achieving homosexual pleasure without the inevitable accompaniment of fear, guilt and self-hatred'.[6] The whole tenor of Meyers's chapter on *Dorian Gray* is that Wilde's novel clumsily betrays what for him is the poisoned well of gay sexual experience, whilst it is in the process of attempting to establish the opposite. He insists on seeing this as a book about 'the damned wasteland of Sodom',[7] that is, gay experience.

A more appropriate way of looking at the excesses and debaucheries of Dorian Gray, and indeed of Byron's characters (if not Byron himself), is the deliberate, proudly perverse owning to the titles conferred by society. Just as derogatory terms ('queer', 'nigger' and so on) have, famously, been adopted by their referents, in a defiant recognition of the challenge, and in an awareness of the kind of society in which they live and the sort of treatment that they can expect to receive, and have in this way placed the situation always to the fore in their minds, so the characters of Wilde and Byron take up an attitude the essence of which is something like this: 'society has, with arbitrary and cruel power, branded me as evil. It expects of me nothing good. Very well. I will live up to this enforced reputation, will make society rue its rejection of me by taking a furious revenge. I will become what they thought I already was.' This is a well-known psychological disposition which, *mutatis mutandis,* affects many social groups. In the present study, it is at its most extreme expression in the life and writings of Jean Genet.

A second literary stimulus for Wilde was the doctrine of aestheticism, and particularly those expressions of it which he found in the work of Georges Huysmans and Walter Pater. The first of these had published a novel called *Against Nature* and Wilde stated after the publication of *Dorian Gray* that the work he was thinking of when he invented the 'poisonous' book with the yellow cover read by Gray was *Against Nature*. Pater's influence came through his notorious conclusion to *Studies in the History of the Renaissance* in which he developed the idea that not morality but sensation should be the true basis of human fulfilment. (Pater later claimed to have been seriously misunderstood, and was alarmed at thus apparently encouraging hedonism.) Thus, for example, 'Art comes to you proposing frankly to bring nothing but the highest quality to your moments as they pass, and simply for those moments' sake' and 'To burn always with this hard, gem-like flame, to maintain this ecstasy, is success in life.'[8] His later novel, *Marius the Epicurean* (1885), has marked similarities to Wilde's; in particular, both novels emphasise the central importance of spiritual development and sensibility, and by comparison the relative unimportance of public events in the observable world. Just as Pater constrasts plagues and earthquakes with the events in Marius' mind, so later Wilde was to present Gray as someone who could retain his equanimity in the face of the suicide of the woman he supposedly loves.

Aestheticism was seen as a serious threat because it undermined one of the basic assumptions of nineteenth century (not to speak of earlier) readers. This was that literature was essentially concerned with moral questions; that individual novels and poems advocated and deplored (not necessarily crudely or explicitly, of course), moved readers to sympathy with the good and detestation of the bad. Behind Wilde was the literary tradition of Fanny Price and Mary Crawford, of Dorothea and Casaubon, Farfrae and Henchard, Slope and Mrs Proudie, Uriah Heap and David Copperfield – in the portrayal of all of whom there is a central preoccupation with moral values. Wilde was to parody the moral approach in *The Importance of Being Earnest*, in which the stuffy governess, Miss Prism, describes her own unpublished novel: 'The good ended happily, and the bad unhappily. That is what Fiction means.'[9]

Wilde frequently denounced the didactic in literature. He claimed that 'books that try to prove anything' should not be read at all.[10] Beauty and style were more important than moral codes: 'I look forward to the time when aesthetics will take the place of ethics, when the sense of beauty will be the dominant law of life.'[11] Specifically referring to the novel, he said: 'I am quite incapable of understanding how any work of art can be criticised from a moral standpoint. . . . I wrote this book [*Dorian Gray*] entirely for my own pleasure'; and in the Preface to the novel, he wrote: 'No artist has ethical sympathies. An ethical sympathy in an artist is an unpardonable mannerism of style.'[12] Much of this was naïve or even hypocritical, as he was stressing the moral importance of *Dorian Gray* at different times but no less emphatically.

The contradiction – leaving aside for the moment the plausible explanation which is simply based on an acceptance of the contradictory nature of human beings – might be explained in this way. Writers and their supporters frequently use the term 'moral' lazily to mean two quite separate things, now one and now the other, creating confusion. The first meaning refers to the accepted codes of polite society and the second meaning refers to the putatively 'genuine' morality (often the opposite of the first, in terms of content) supported by the writer in question. The history of censorship is packed with examples – Nabokov's *Lolita*, Selby's *Last Exit to Brooklyn*, Lawrence's *Lady Chatterley's Lover*, and so on – of supposed immorality denounced by the works' attackers (first definition) and supposed morality of the same work (second definition) claimed by supporters. It appears that the interest of both parties is best served by leaving the distinction blurred.

Wilde's version of aestheticism, as articulated in *Dorian Gray*, involves the idea that 'doing good' is cowardly, that giving in to temptation, rather than resisting it, is the truly courageous act: 'Conscience and cowardice are really the same things, Basil'; 'The only way to get rid of a temptation is to yield to it. Resist it, and your soul grows sick with longing for the things it has forbidden to itself, with desire for what its monstrous laws have made monstrous and unlawful.'[13] Notice in this last quotation that it is not society on this occasion which is being blamed for making 'monstrous laws', but the individual soul. This is a recognition that, whatever the exterior oppressions in the public world, consenting to live under their domain is not an inevitable decision. The existentialist individual must take responsibility for his life without seeking to blame outside forces for his acts. In this sense, Wilde continues the existentialist theme evident in Byron and in many of the writers after him, studied in this book.

The whole theory expounded in *Dorian Gray* concerning morality is rendered more or less absurd on an intellectual level because of the confusion in the use of terms. For example, it cannot be good/better to subjugate ethics to aesthetics when 'good/better' are ethical terms, which means that preferring aesthetics is an ethical act. These confusions emerge frequently: 'Modern morality consists in accepting the standard of one's age. I consider that for any man of culture to accept the standard of his age is a form of the grossest immorality.'[14]

It is often considered inappropriate to cavil at the intellectual absurdities of a literary work, on the basis that such a complaint is based on a flawed view of what literature attempts. On this view, the whole emotional effect should be considered, and no attempt should be made to see the work in question as a disguised intellectual thesis. It does seem to me that *Dorian Gray* does offer itself in part as precisely that, and that such criticisms as I have made are at least *a priori* valid. Nevertheless, we need not dwell on this.

Byron's hatred of cant, of disguise and pretence, was of course based on his own practice of precisely those things, albeit in a different way. Wilde is in the same position: forced to conceal a central aspect of his identity (his sexual orientation) through elaborate symbols of decadent living (involving gardens, fine tapestries and brocades), he virulently denounces the hypocrisies of his age. The book is filled with satirical observations on the behaviour of the English ruling class. He insists in the Preface: 'The nineteenth century dislike of Realism is the rage of Caliban seeing his own face in a glass.'[15]

Rejecting the mainstream involves choosing an alternative. For Byron it is, crudely, adventure. For Genet it is self-abasement and revenge-crime. For Williams, Forster and Isherwood, it is polite protest and indignation. Wilde's choice in *Dorian Gray* is decadent hedonism. Having rejected the moral significance of literature, books are placed on the same level as curtains, flowers and exquisite meals. The opening of Chapter One conveys the self-indulgence involved:

> The studio was filled with the rich odour of roses, and when the light summer wind stirred amidst the trees of the garden there came through the open door the heavy scent of the lilac, or the more delicate perfume of the pink-flowering thorn.
>
> From the corner of the divan of Persian saddlebags on which he was lying, smoking, as was his custom, innumerable cigarettes, Lord Henry Wotton could just catch the gleam of the honey-sweet and honey-coloured blossoms of a laburnum . . . (p. 1.)

Byron and Wilde, then, are both rebels: in their writing, and equally, in their lives. They insist courageously on turning away from the spurious 'democracy' of the mob and its mindless conformity. At the same time, they are cautious and fearful. Now they stand on the soapbox, now they cower in the shadows. In the end, both literally fled their country. These contrarities of resistance and fear, of proclaiming and hiding, taken with the existentialist motif in the works, are to be recurring themes in the gay writing of the twentieth century.

3

The Poems of Constantine Cavafy

Constantine Cavafy (1863–1933) was the ninth and last child of his parents. Apart from seven years in England, between the ages of nine and sixteen (spent away from home because of his family business interests) most of his life was passed in Alexandria, where he spent his working life in the Egyptian Ministry of Public Works. He was considered especially useful there because of his skill in foreign languages. (His English was particularly good.) His life was generally uneventful in the public sense; privately, if the poems are as autobiographical as most readers assume, it was full of intense experiences. A number of unpublished notes found after his death show that he suffered from a guilt arising from what he saw as his relentless autoeroticism. He kept in touch with certain literary figures of the time, most famously E. M. Forster, whom he knew for twenty years.

His poems were not published during his lifetime, but circulated by Cavafy himself to a select group of readers in constantly revised folders. It is widely, and in my view correctly, thought that his poems only reach maturity with the author's arrival at middle age. His enormous reputation accrued after his death.

[Note on the translations: the poems quoted below have all been translated by Cyril Winters. Cavafy's poems were written in demotic Greek. The sexual daring of many of the poems is sometimes a little misleading, as in demotic Greek pronouns can be used which do not indicate gender, although English translations now always give 'he', 'him', etc.]

there is no other garden like love

(Cavafy, *Good and Bad Weather*)

Regret, doleful memory, occasional twinges of conscience about homosexuality, and an obsession with time and with the ageing process, all inform Cavafy's work. In general, however, his poems celebrate love unapologetically and enthusiastically. They are charged with erotic force and saturated in the history and present state of his beloved Alexandria.

From the start, Cavafy is the loner. One of the earliest poems insists on a superior separateness from what V. S. Naipaul is later to call the 'infies' (inferiors):[1]

I don't ask whether or not I'm content.
But I'm always pleased to remember one thing:
that in the huge addition – that addition of theirs that I hate –
which is so numerous, I am not one
of the many units there. I was not counted
in the total sum. And the pleasure of knowing this, is sufficient.

In 'As Much As You Can' the speaker, using, as so frequently in Cavafy, the imperative mood, tells us not to cheapen our lives with too much contact with the world, with its silliness and tediousness. The implied message is that we should savour the rare, the worthwhile, which is frequently art.

So it is that in another early poem, 'Artificial Flowers', Cavafy rejects 'real flowers' in favour of the artificial. He does not want perishable, everyday beauty, but the timeless fashioning of art. And, 'If they have no scent, we will provide fragrance . . .' (We know the debate already: the poems of D. H. Lawrence on the benefits of the short-lived, versus the Yeats of 'Byzantium'.)

The emphasis on the artificial is *fin de siècle* in sentiment. It is literally that too (the 'early' poems come from 1886–1904). We shall therefore not be surprised to find, throughout Cavafy's work, a Wildean set of values: about defying the canons of conduct and taste in a loutish culture, about refusing to feel guilty about sexual pleasure, about retaining personal integrity, tenderness, a kind of softness. And about courage.

Courage requires an acceptance of individual responsibility. No passing the buck; no 'bad faith'. In 'The City', a character seeks out a new city in order to find a better life. The speaker points out to him that, if you've destroyed your life in one place, you have destroyed it everywhere in the world. Moving to a new place is dishonestly denying the real cause of the malaise, which is not in the city but within oneself. 'Ithaka' has a similar idea in a powerful but altogether different kind of metaphor: Ulysses, says the poem's speaker, won't encounter Poseidon and the Cyclops unless they are in his soul already. Environments can be overcome by the imagination. Nothing is, but thinking makes it so. It is a crucial part of this poem that the journeying is important, the destination is not.

In 'The God Abandons Antony', Cavafy's speaker again exhorts courage. Mark Antony hears the processional music of Alexandria, the city he must leave for ever. But there must be no histrionic wailing. Depth of feeling is vulgarised by anything raucous; a brave, tranquil decorum (such as Genet describes the fedayeen of the PLO as having, before their fatal missions) is proper:

> go determinedly to the window
> and listen with great feeling
> but not with the obsequious begging of the coward . . .

This note is sounded again, with the same unemcumbered directness, in 'Thermopylae', a hymn of praise to the nobility, generosity and courage of those warriors fighting (many of them) in the knowledge of their own imminent defeat and death.

Bertrand Russell says in the second volume of his autobiography that he could never love any woman who lacked courage; he feels, starkly, that there can be no moral order without it. For Cavafy too, it is perhaps the pre-eminent virtue. Without it, the mob rules. For injustice to prevail, it is only necessary for just men to say nothing. Cavafy's adherence to this maxim is passionate.

As if to hammer home the need for resignation in the face of adversity or the unexpected, Cavafy repeatedly seizes on historical moments of sudden reversal: the Greeks at Thermopylae about to be slain ('Thermopylae'); the murderers' footsteps creeping up to the still youthful Nero's bedroom ('The Footsteps'); Artemidoros' warning to Caesar on his way to the senate ('The Ides of March').

Moral courage, the sustaining power of art, the rejection of the crowd; these are where we start. As we shall see, in the love poetry they are always there, implied or made explicit.

In an early poem, Cavafy presents us with a dialogue between a poet and his muse. The poet wishes to 'sing of noble sentiments' but he finds that virtue and glory are mere dreams. There is discouragement wherever he looks. The real world is soiled; it seems to make a nonsense of anything written in a celebratory style. It seems, in fact, as if joyous poets are liars. The reply of the muse consists of sentiments which inform the whole of Cavafy's work:

> Poet, you are no liar. The world that you imagine,
> is the real one. The melodies of the harp
> Alone know truth, and in this life
> they can be our only true guides.
>
> ('The Poet and the Muse')

Cavafy, the bulk of whose work was written after this poem, heeds this sentiment. Anticipating Proust, he insists on the supremacy of the mind and its imagination, over the sordid so-called realities of life.

The subject matter of Cavafy's poems can be divided into two. First, there are poems dealing with ideas of history and place, especially historical anecdotes or potted histories or vignettes of (often aristocratic) figures from the ancient world. Ancient Alexandria is evoked repeatedly, so much so that for many Cavafy commentators, the city (in which Cavafy spent most of his life) becomes almost a living character in its own right.[2] The second general category of poems is that dealing with love – love in all its meanings, from selfless solicitude to casual sexual encounters, from the heart's longing to the frankly erotic. In this chapter I shall be dealing primarily with these sexual poems, but where appropriate I shall also discuss poems from the first group. There is, of course, considerable interchange: poems about Alexandria, or ancient historical events and persons, frequently deal centrally with love.

Typically, Cavafy's poems are of the past; they do not celebrate present pleasure, but significant memory of it. At the heart of Cavafy's notion of human being is the Proustian idea of transcendence through memory and art. That is to say, the recollection (in memory), or the recreation (through art), or both these processes together, transform the original experience, making it live again but at the same time making it live in a different way. For both Proust and Cavafy, this remaking, which is often the act of writing itself, is frequently more valuable and intense as a lived experience than the events recollected.

The act of recollection has two distinct strands: the details which are recalled from one's past, and one's present attitude towards them. These two aspects can never be separated in the act of recollection, and Cavafy's poems contain them both. As the speaker's mood changes in these poems, so does the content and interrelationship of these two categories. There is thus no objective memory in the poems, but rather a highly varied and subjective series of glimpses of the unfolded years.

You will see that I am speaking of Cavafy's poems as self-evidently a coherent group rather than a motley collection. Indeed, it is often said that the poems, which to some readers can appear (especially in translation) to be somewhat inconsequential when taken individually, acquire a resonance and force when taken as a group, with various echoes and repetitions gradually building up into, as the process of reading continues, an identifiably unified whole. This coherence is also evinced in the fact not only that there is a return time and again to the same limited number of themes, but also in the fact that the sensibilities of the various speakers in the poems are very similar. The *personae* do change, in terms of identity (for example, from an old man to a young one, from a historical character from the ancient world to a sleazy youth from contemporary Alexandria), and in terms of viewpoint (now defiant, now full of remorse), but there are only a limited number of fixed types.

A frequent type is the unabashed sensualist, whose days of pleasure are over. His concern is the savouring anew of past delights, either his own or those of others. For example, 'Two Young Men, 23 to 24 Years Old' tells of a young man waiting disconsolately for three hours in a gradually emptying cafe for his lover, broke, and worried about the 'immorality of his way of life'. Then his lover appears and the boredom disappears. The lover has won a fortune at cards, and they decide to give themselves to pleasure:

> Filled at this moment with pleasure and strength, emotion and beauty,

they took themselves, not back home to their respectable families
(who didn't want to see them anyway)
but to a place well-known to them, and very special,
a house of notoriety, and they took a bedroom,
and ordered expensive drinks, and continued their drinking.

And when they had done with their expensive drinks,
and at this stage it was almost four o'clock
They gave themselves happily to love.

This poem contains two common Cavafy themes: first, the seedy surroundings which give a piquancy to the sexual experience; secondly, the moral uncertainty which sometimes rears its head. We shall say something of both these ideas.

First, the sordidness. Cavafy returns over and over to details of cheap rooms, dirty cafes, tatty clothes. In 'One Night', this contrast constitutes the chief meaning of the poem: the irony that love flourishes in unpromising and 'unromantic' locations and circumstances, and this in turn establishes the extraordinary resilience and power of love to overcome obstacles. Blooms can flourish in the desert:

> The room was cheap and common
> Tucked away over a low-life taverna.
> You could see the alley from the window,
> Dirty and cramped.

In 'The Photograph', the speaker lingers over a pornographic photograph, of the kind sold surreptitiously in the street, whilst the vendor keeps a weather eye open for the police. The life of the man photographed is imagined as cheap and vulgar, but in spite of this a rich enchantment hangs over him:

> Despite all this, and more, for me you retain
> the sort of face one sees in a dream, a body
> made and intended for the Greek sort of pleasure . . .

This combination of low-life and breathtaking beauty occurs again in 'Days of 1908'. Unemployed, and making ends meet with a bit of gambling, the man described in this poem embodies the typical Cavafy youth: under the dreary suit, he is ravishingly beautiful in his nakedness:

> Your view has preserved him
> as he was when he took off those unworthy clothes,
> that mended underwear, threw it all aside,
> and stood stark naked, impeccably handsome, a miracle –
> his hair uncombed, swept back,
> his limbs a little tanned
> from his morning nakedness at the baths and on the beach.

The tatty clothes and impoverished background serve to highlight the physical charms. It is also plain that the experience of sex in Cavafy's poems is an escape from, and a kind of denial of, the poverty in which it takes place.

Cavafy's evocation of sordidness is sometimes linked with the financial exploitation of sexual attractiveness. We have seen one example of this already in 'The Photograph', but it is usually prostitution rather than posing for pictures which is involved. Typical of this group of poems is 'Days of 1909, '10, and '11'. The subject wears shabby clothes and works for an ironmonger; his shoes are torn and his hands filthy with rust and oil. Sometimes, wandering in the evenings, he takes a fancy to an expensive tie or a shirt, and then 'he'd sell his body for a few shillings'. The idea of sex for sale is already a tantalising notion. It is perhaps more so if the seller is not habitually prostituting himself (which might indicate an offhand or indifferent, certainly an unenthusiastic love-making) but someone who does such a thing occasionally, on a whim (suggesting a more daring youth and therefore a more exciting sexual tryst for the punter). Secondly, the context of financial payment has two corollaries: a depersonalised if not actually anonymous sexual exchange (in itself very often highly valued by the sexual participant) and an enhanced sense of power and control over the payee. After all, one cannot easily direct the bedroom conduct of an unpaid lover.

Sometimes, Cavafy creates an ambiguous situation whereby the boy who is selling himself is neither coldly mercenary nor indifferent to payment for sexual favours; he is fond of his current protector but on the other hand, he cannot easily decline higher offers. In 'Lovely White Flowers', two 'friends' sit at a cafe and one tells the other that he (the former) must transfer his allegiance to somebody else because that other person has promised to buy him new clothes. Cavafy also presents us with the sexual pride of the man who has managed to hold on to the loyalty of a beautiful youth without payment, out of love. The speaker in 'In the Tavernas' has now lost his friend and is now giving up his life, despairingly, to 'sordid debauchery', but:

> The one thing that consoles me,
> like lasting beauty or perfume,
> the thing that I can cling onto still, is this: Tamides,
> most exquisite of young men, was mine for two years,
> mine completely and not for a house or a villa on the Nile.

Thus, Cavafy records both the experiences and sensations of those who pay for sex, and those who take pride in not doing so. He also represents the lifestyle of the brothel habitué, sometimes exciting and fulfilling, sometimes desperate and empty.

Thus, the situations conventionally called 'sordid' are, in Cavafy's poetry, often exciting as well as sad.

After the theme of seediness, the second major theme that we noted in 'Two Young Men, 23 to 24 Years Old' was moral uncertainty. In this poem, one of the young men is not at all happy about the 'immorality' of his life. It is hardly surprising that we should find this sentiment on a number of occasions in Cavafy. He was writing long before the time when hetero-supremacist views had lost any of their footing. Thus, in the poem 'In Despair', we read of 'the tainted form of sexual pleasure' and in many of the historical poems, the youthful protagonists are fighting (unsuccessfully) against their gay sexual desires in a way which the tone of the speaker suggests is virtuous.

On the other hand, there are far more poems plainly attacking the tired orthodoxies of sexual morality. In a very early example, 'An Old Man', we have described an old man who led a life of respectability and self-denial in order to conform to the morality of his society and now, in his decline, bitterly regrets 'how little he enjoyed the years/When he had strength and wit, and vigour':

> He knows he's very old: he can feel it.
> Yet the time when he was young is fresh in the mind.

How recent that all appears; as though only yesterday.
He remembers how Prudence tricked him
how he always believed, so foolishly,
that cheat who said: 'Do it another day. You have plenty of time.'
He remembers impulses checked, the pleasure
he sacrificed. The memory of every lost opportunity
now mocks his meaningless prudence.

In 'Che Fece . . . Il Gran Rifuto', we hear of the moment when we have to give to life 'the great Yes or the great No' and he who gives the conventional answer – in this context, he who says 'no' to a life of sensuality – finds that that 'no' ('the right no' as far as received opinion is concerned) 'drags him down all his life'. In 'Days of 1896', the speaker records that the protagonist, in his life of sexual indulgence, put his body before his honour, and then concludes:

. . . But society,
in its bigotry, had all its values wrong.

The radical nature of Cavafy's view on these matters is encapsulated in 'Growing in Spirit', given here in its entirety:

He who aspires to grow in spirit
will have to go beyond conformity and respect.
He'll go along with some laws, certainly,
but for the most part he'll reject
both laws and customs, and go beyond
the established, inadequate norms.
Sensual pleasures will have much to teach him.
He won't be frightened of being destructive;
half the house will have to come down.
In this way he'll learn wisdom virtuously.

Taken together, these anti-convention poems are putting forward a view which is quite different from the orthodox wing of gay liberation of the 1970s, which can perhaps be expressed in the formula: 'we are equal, we are proud, and we want a (conventional) place in the sun in the existing society'. Rather, he says (anticipating Genet) something like this:

> Mainstream society is suffocatingly conventional; as a gay man, I accept, indeed (sometimes) enthusiastically embrace the 'outsider', 'perverse' status accorded to my identity by such a contemptible society. My sexuality, and its expression in physical actions, is therefore a kind of revolt against that society, having social and political significance far beyond the sexual. In fucking men, I do not merely break a specific taboo; I question the authority, the reasonableness, the sanity of those formulating such taboos. My experience of my sexual identity, and its rejection by straight society, has led me to see the connections between conventions of personal sexual behaviour and political oppression in general.'

We should remember that one of Cavafy's earliest poems ('1896') presents us with a simple parable of how society can encroach, *unnoticed*, on the unwary, until we find that we are outflanked and the battle is lost. Those 'who prattle about morality' ('Theatre of Sidon') are the enemy. Religion, especially Christianity and Judaism, are pernicious. In 'Myris', the speaker tells of how he fled from the house of his beloved Myris, now dead, before his memory 'could be polluted by Christianity'. The cost of personal freedom is eternal vigilance against the seeping and insidious inroads of orthodoxy:

> Without consideration, or pity, or shame,
> they've built thick high walls all round me.
> And now I sit in here feeling desperate.
> I can think of nothing but this fate, which gnaws at my mind –
> because I had so much to do outside.
> When they were building the walls, why didn't I take notice!
> But I never heard a sound from the builders,
> Imperceptibly they've shut me off from the outside world.
>
> ('Walls')

Part of the unconventionality in Cavafy's picture of sexual relationships is the relatively unanguished acceptance of the brevity of love and desire. Brevity is not necessarily seen as negative, but as something innate in relationships. He is articulating the Lawrentian view[3] that love blossoms like a flower and like a flower it should be allowed to wither and die in due season, without artificial means being employed to resuscitate it:

> It wouldn't have lasted long anyhow.
> My experience over the years tells me that.
> Nevertheless, Fate did end it rather suddenly.
> That wonderful life was soon finished.
> Yet how strong the scents were,
> what a wonderful bed we lay in,
> And what pleasures we gave our bodies.
> ('In the Evening')

There is resentment here that the relationship has ended ('rather suddenly') but there is also acceptance. We get the same sort of mix in 'Before Time Changed Them', here given in full:

> They were both full of grief at their parting.
> They hadn't wanted it: circumstances dictated it.
> The need to earn a living forced one of them
> to go far away – New York or Canada.
> Their love wasn't, of course, what it had been;
> the attraction between them had begun to cool,
> the attraction and the excitement.
> But to be separated wasn't what they wanted.
> It was circumstance. Or perhaps Fate
> appeared, an artist, and now decided to separate them,
> before their feeling withered, before time altered them:
> the one will always remain for the other what he was,
> the handsome young man of twenty-four.

In Cavafy, it is not merely that the most exciting and impassioned relationships are brief; we also see that their end can be poignantly sudden. 'The Afternoon Sun' concludes:

> . . . One afternoon we parted at four o'clock,
> just for a week . . . And then –
> that week became forever.

The emphasis on the brevity of love underlines an important aspect of Cavafy's poetry, which is his preoccupation with time.

In an early poem, 'Come Back' (1912), the speaker apostrophises the sensation of love itself. He asks that this sensation come back to him. The poem is short (eight lines) and, as this outline suggests, highly abstract. We are not introduced to the character of the speaker or the people associated with his longing; rather, Cavafy, as in a Chinese watercolour, uses an extremely spare and minimalist set of expressions to convey the intensity of the experience, rather than its quality or attributes. It reminds us strongly of Ezra Pound's 'Liu Che',[4] a poem of mourning, in which the eponymous deceased is not described at all, but evoked through details (the dryness of leaves, the rustling of silk) which convey the desolation of the bereaved one. That is to say, the poem indirectly comments on the person Liu Che by describing the void left by her death. The speaker in 'Come Back', like Count Orsino in *Twelfth Night*, is in love with the idea of love and its attendant experiences. The identity of the beloved is hardly relevant. The poem is an admittedly extreme example of Cavafy's tendency, in memory poems, towards spareness.

'Long Ago', written two years later (1914), is self-absorbed in the same way as 'Come Back', but refinements have been added:

> I'd like to describe this memory,
> but it is now so faded – hardly anything is left –
> because it took place so long ago, in my youth.
>
> At night, a skin as though made of jasmine . . .
> that August evening – was it August? –
> I can hardly remember the eyes: blue, I think they were . . .
> Or was it September
> That's right, they were blue; as blue as sapphire.

Unlike 'Come Back', this poem is typographically fragmentary. The dots and the dashes interrupting the lines convey the ruptured and disordered process of recalling the past. This feature and the uncertainty of the speaker as to details – was it August or not? – give the impression of a poem being written simultaneously with the speaker undergoing the experience of the feelings it describes. This is particularly obvious in the final two lines, where the speaker is correcting and annotating as he goes along. We are still entitled to call this writing spare, but here details do matter. The point about the colour of the eyes is that, out of such apparently minor features, a vast mental edifice of longing, recollection, wistfulness and confusion has grown up. There are therefore two subjects of the poem: the past itself, and the nature of present emotions concerning it. This double feature occurs in most of the memory poems. In them, we usually find out more about the experience of recollection than the specific events which give rise to them.

'Grey' (1917) is also short and fragmentary, and based on the evocation of sparse details: here, a pair of grey eyes. The speaker acknowledges that the eyes will have lost their charm with the years – 'that lovely face will have lost its charm' – so he calls upon memory to bring back the recollection of what they were like in the past, so as to facilitate a general recollection of the whole sensation of the relationship. And there is a new note here, the urgency. The last three lines convey a speaker needing the past as a consolation for a dismal present:

> Memory, keep them as they were.
> And, memory, whatever you can bring back of that love,
> bring it back tonight.

In 'Since Nine O'Clock' (1918) the speaker has been at home since nine, unable to get down to reading because he is haunted by the memory of the 'closed, scented rooms,/of past passion'. Here, memory is itself a force disrupting the life of the speaker, preventing him from getting on with everyday living. One of Cavafy's ways of insisting on the excitement of sexual memories, and sexuality itself, is to make reading its opposite. What is supposed to be the tediously intellectual is counterpointed against the 'animal' instinct. This idea is even clearer in the masturbation poem, 'He Had Come There to Read', in which the protagonist, although 'utterly devoted to books', succumbs to Eros and abandons his history and poetry books (books, we note, of especial interest to Cavafy himself) for a masturbation session. 'Since Nine O'Clock' ends with:

> Half past twelve: how the hours have gone by.
> Half past twelve: how the years have gone by.

and we register here a habitual sentiment. That is to say, the poem speaks of one day's experience, but we read it as typical of a recurring and regular pattern. This is merely one occasion, but it somehow contains the desperate sameness of all the rest.

The distressing invasion of these involuntary thoughts – producing a mournful restlessness – is a constant Cavafy theme. There is a sweetness to them too, of course; one might say that the poems' poignancy is precisely because of this blending of regret (because the events are past) and delight (because the events were at least experienced). There is a further consideration – that the articulation of this melancholy in poetry is itself therapeutic – which is something we shall consider in greater detail below.

Cavafy also employs the *carpe diem* theme. (The Latin words mean 'seize the day'; in such poems the addressee and/or speaker is being urged to enjoy life while there is still time. The most famous example is Marvell's 'To His Coy Mistress'.) This theme can be represented by an early poem, 'I Went' (1913):

> I didn't hold back, but wholly abandoned myself, and went
> to those pleasures that were half real,
> and half created in my own mind;
> I went into the brilliant night,
> and drank strong wine in the same manner
> as the champions of pleasure drink.

There is defiance here, a recognition that the sensible middle-aged paths of prudence are being boisterously rejected. And there is of course an exuberance in that very defiance, a snatching at pleasure while it is still possible. We can see two further points of interest in this poem: first, the insistence in line 3 that pleasure is partly imaginative, not something merely physiological; secondly, the desire to emulate the champions. This unashamedly vain-glorious streak in Cavafy's poems recurs frequently.

The memory of an erotic encounter, written down in a poem, can serve as some kind of palliative against the anguished knowledge that the incident characterises a way of life no longer possible because of change and ageing. In 'To Remain', the speaker remembers a sexual encounter between himself and another man behind the wooden partition of a tavern. It is a hot July day, the waiter is asleep, the men's clothes are already half-opened, and, leaving them half-opened, they enjoy each other. The poem ends:

. . . here was a vision
that has come to me over twenty-six years
and now comes to rest in these lines.

'Very Seldom' tells the story of an old man, physically maimed by the passing of years and yet, in one way, holding on to youth. The sensual poetry that he wrote is stimulating the young to erotic fantasies; their lust operates through his eyes. The art of poetry thus provides a vicarious satisfaction. In 'Their Beginning', a pair of furtive lovers is described as moving down the street, wary lest observers infer what they have been doing. But in contrast to this present apprehension is the wonderful poetry which will be inspired by this sexual encounter in the future:

How the artist's life has gained from this!
Tomorrow, the next day, or years later,
Strong lines will be written that had their inspiration here.

In the 'Melancholy of Jason Kleander', the speaker talks of the process of his own ageing as like the action of a ruthless knife. He turns to the 'art of poetry' as to a soothing drug, which will, temporarily, relieve the pain. These two ideas – art as a transcendent drug whose effect is regrettably temporary – are of course famously present in the odes of John Keats. In 'Ode on Melancholy', Keats opens the poem by exhorting the reader *not* to take wine or drugs to soothe the soul's melancholy, but rather to hug it to oneself as a kind of perverse pleasure. The opening stanzas of 'Ode to a Nightingale' similarly involve the idea of taking wine, hemlock and an opiate in order to escape 'The weariness, the fever, and the fret' of everyday life. In the poem, the speaker rejects these substances which promise oblivion, because it is poetry itself which will take him away from 'reality' into a reverie based on a sympathy with the nightingale – a reverie which is short-lived and ends as the bird flies away. Both Cavafy and Keats make it clear that the process of writing the poem, which has for subject matter some mournful recollection of lost pleasures (Cavafy) or a lament on the sordid nature of existence (Keats), is itself a palliative to those pangs. The creative process of writing is therapeutic, counteracting the source of the poets' anguish.

Neither Keats or Cavafy (unlike Proust) felt that art could fully compensate for what was disappointing about the 'real' world – it was something of a delirious and temporary compensation. This half-heartedness is illustrated in Cavafy's 'Half an Hour', here given in full:

> I never slept with you and I don't suppose
> I ever will. A couple of words, an approach,
> as at the bar yesterday – nothing more.
> I admit that it's sad. But those of us dedicated to Art,
> sometimes with a mental intensity
> can create pleasure that seems almost physical –
> but of course only for a short time.
> That's how in the bar yesterday –
> helped, thank goodness, by drink –
> I had half an hour that was completely erotic.
> And I think you knew
> and deliberately stayed slightly longer.
> That was certainly needed.
> Because with all the imagination,
> and all the magical alcohol,
> I needed actually to see your lips as well,
> and needed your body close to me.

In Cavafy's work, enormous importance is attached to physical beauty, especially in the love poems. In 'Tomb of Evrion', the dead man is described as a historian, theologian and a philosopher, but:

> we've lost what was truly valuable: his physique –
> like a vision of Apollo

'At the Cafe Door' records the speaker catching a glimpse of a beautiful man in a doorway, 'as though Eros himself had made it, with all his skill'. The statue of Endymion ('Before the Statue of Endymion'), the poet Ammonis ('For Ammonis, Who Died At 29, In 610') and the brother-in-law of Herod the Great ('Aristovoulos') are further examples. In the case of the last two, tragically premature deaths add to the sexual piquancy, for it is as though the physical desirability embodied in these men is not allowed by death to decay but is ended at the zenith.

The overriding importance of physical beauty in Cavafy's celebrations of the erotic is a problematic one for modern readers. It is one thing – and Cavafy assuredly does this with vigour and passion – to celebrate the body and the pleasures of sexuality, especially when the poems have been written and are now and have in the past been read, in the context of societies which hypocritically or mean-mindedly denounce such pleasures out of perverse jealousy or some harmful dogma (usually Christianity or Judaism in Cavafy's work). But it is certainly another thing to exalt beauty to such an extent, to confer on it such a premium, that it is represented as an indispensable attribute for a successful human life.

In Cavafy's poems, we notice a clear effort to de-romanticise relationships. In 'Lovely White Flowers', there is a decidedly mercenary aspect to the relationship described. Cavafy avoids the facile assumption that relationships will be either loving or mercenary, and is able to tell us of couples who experience something of both. Here, the central character, described by the speaker in the third person, loses his lover because the latter has been offered better inducements from another man. These amount to two suits and some silk handkerchiefs. The first man scrapes together enough money to as it were 'buy back' the lover, and is successful. The point is that the lover, though prepared to change allegiance for mercenary reasons, is also genuinely attached to his first love and delighted to resume the relationship with him. There were 'strong feelings between them'.

The poem ends with the death of the lover, beautiful in his twenty two years as he lies in his coffin which is bedecked with white flowers. The survivor cannot bear to revisit the cafe where they used to spend time together without feeling 'a knife in his heart'. In almost all the love poems, there is this sort of despondency running parallel with the sexual delight; it is as if Cavafy feels a price, and usually a high one, must be paid for the experience of love.

This despondency is apparent in 'Two Young Men, 23 to 24 Years Old', quoted above. It begins as a man waits for hours on end for his lover; he has little money; he has smoked his last cigarette. Suddenly, the situation is transformed by the arrival of the lover, who has won a small fortune at cards, and Cavafy switches dramatically from the depressing to the celebratory. Relationships which are entirely smooth, harmonious, unruptured, safe, are not depicted in Cavafy. Instead, we have a host of problems which, however, are frequently vanquished temporarily in the delirious oblivion of sex.

But there is guilt. In the poem just discussed, the waiting man begins to be worried with doubts about 'the indecent life he was living'. In 'Dangerous Thoughts', a fourth century Syrian student decides to give himself up to lascivious delights and 'the most daring erotic desires' but he can say this to himself because at the same time he is promising himself a reformation. When the time comes, we learn in the last lines: 'I'll recover/my puritan spirit as it was originally.' This guilt – hardly surprising in a poet writing in the early years of this century, when even the poetic evocations of heterosexual sex needed to be circumspect – is found in many Cavafy poems. Its flavour is well rendered by 'He Swears', here quoted in full:

> He swears every now and again to begin a better life
> But when the night arrives, with its own advice
> With its own compromises and prospects
> When night comes with its own sway
> Over a body that desires and demands
> He falls back again, lost, in the same fatal pleasure.

That final phrase suggests that it may be that the sexual experiences are so pleasurable partly because they are forbidden. Some support is given to this view by 'Imenos', in which the speaker talks of corrupt and morbid sexual pleasures being especially intoxicating. They have 'an erotic intensity, unknown to healthiness'. (We are reminded of Genet's defiant longing for debasement and guilt, which for him offered a kind of perverse recognition.)

Wounds, pain and death are part of Cavafy's erotic world. 'The Bandaged Shoulder' describes the speaker tending a man's wound. (Hart Crane and Walt Whitman write of this situation too.) He likes looking at the blood, it is 'a thing of my love'. When the beloved departs, the speaker holds to his lips for a long time a blood-stained, soiled, discarded dressing. The poignancy is in the daring: it is 'disgusting' (to the cool-hearted), and embarrassingly private and intimate, and yet full of the love which wishes to minister, to protect, to nurse.

'In a town of Osroini' tells of a man wounded in a brawl in the local tavern. The speaker finds his beauty enhanced now that his body is wounded. Again, as in the previous poem, it seems to be connected with a greater vulnerability in the situation of the beloved. Lying supine and helpless, or having sustained some injury, places the sufferer in a position of dependence which Cavafy's speakers find sexually exciting. An extreme statement of this is found in 'The Funeral Of Sarpedon'. Patroclus has killed the eponymous subject, and the god Apollo is tending the body. Lovingly, he combs the black hair and spreads out the beautiful limbs:

> And now he looks like a young king, a charioteer
> twenty five or twenty six
> resting himself after winning a race

The sleep/death parallel is of course a literary topos (*Hamlet, Measure for Measure,* John Donne's 'Death be not proud' for example). Here, the simplicity of the image makes it striking. The dead body is sexually arousing, as in 'Lovely White Flowers', but the state of death is also, and simultaneously, enticing. Apart from anything else, the idea of a young death combines the notion of preserved innocence (God takes early to himself the purest of his flock, as Christians frequently say) with a kind of perpetuating of their beauty, now free from the hideous processes (as Cavafy sees it) of ageing.

Sexual love in Cavafy is often secretive, poignant, brief. It can even consume the participant, as in 'Days of 1909, '10, and '11' which describes a beautiful youth working in an ironmongery, filthy in clothes and general appearance, who, because he gives himself to sensuality, is soon 'used up'. What the reader is most likely to remember and cherish about these poems, however, is their enthusiasm for same-sex pleasure, their unambiguous affirmation of the rights of the sensualist:

> What he timidly imagined as a schoolboy
> are now revealed to him. He walks around the streets at night
> involves himself. And rightly (for the sake of our art)
> his hot new blood is devoted to pleasure. His body is

overwhelmed
by sexual intoxication, and his youthful limbs
are entirely given up to this.
Thus does a simple youth
become noteworthy
and this simple boy with fresh, hot blood
journeys through the elevated realms of Poetry.
('In Transit', quoted entire)

4

E. M. Forster: *Maurice*

E. M. Forster (1879–1970) was brought up by his mother in Hertfordshire and later Kent, his father having died when he was a baby. He read Classics and History at Cambridge, and began to teach Latin at a working men's club in Bloomsbury, London. He travelled widely in Italy, Austria and Greece, and went to Germany as a childrens' tutor. His first novel, Where Angels Fear to Tread, *was published in 1905, but only with* Howards End *(1910), the third novel, did he begin to have commercial success. He went to India for two protracted visits (1912 and 1921) and in 1924 published his most successful work,* A Passage to India. *He cultivated literary acquaintances with Forrest Reid, Constantine Cavafy, Edward Carpenter and J. R. Ackerley, the last of whom became a life-long friend. Only in middle age did he begin any kind of sex life, which was mostly with tough working-class types, whom he preferred. His closest friend in the second part of his life was the policeman Bob Buckingham, whom he met in 1929.*

In the second part of his life he left behind novel writing for other activities: lecturing abroad, involving himself in PEN and the National Council for Civil Liberties, of which he was twice president, and broadcasting. He was given rooms at King's College, Cambridge and elected an honorary fellow there. He appeared as a defence witness in the 1960 obscenity trial of Lawrence's Lady Chatterley's Lover. *He was the classic liberal: he hated oppression and unfairness, but supported most of the élitist institutions (including Cambridge) which fostered them. He is admired by homosexual reactionaries like the novelist Francis King (columnist for the far-right* Spectator *magazine) and despised by gay radicals for staying in the closet even after 1967, when his coming out could have been so beneficial in the struggle for equality.*

Maurice[1] was written, for the most part, between 1913 and 1914, and published after Forster's death in 1971. (He worked on revisions in 1919, 1932 and 1959–60.) His decision to withhold publication was partly a result of doubts about its being dated, and partly the fear of the uproar a homosexual novel could cause, even as late as the 1960s, coming from the pen of such a celebrated author.

When 'dated' is used of novels in this way, what is being suggested is not simply that the social concerns and background have changed to so marked an extent that a story set in the past may appear quaint or lack immediacy of relevance. Rather, the suggestion is that the novel fails to transcend its particular time, that it lacks a universal dimension which will appeal to readers irrespective of the setting. Novels which are dated in this sense are therefore rarely very distinguished. One approach to *Maurice* is to enquire whether it is dated in this sense.

We hear early on that 'No one could be deeply interested in the Halls' (p. 12). A link is established quickly between respectability and tedium. This is symbolised by the stockbroking career of Maurice Hall himself; it is secure, worthy, class-bound and above all, safe. The human cost of possessing oneself of that safety – with its attendant privileges, servants and security – is, at the very least, a kind of radical moral stupidity:

> I've had to do with the poor too,' said Maurice, taking a piece of cake, 'but I can't worry over them. One must give them a leg up for the sake of the country generally, that's all. They haven't our feelings. They don't suffer as we should in their place. (p. 154)

It is the sort of stupidity recognised as actually indicating 'safety', for we read immediately following the above lines: 'Anne looked disapproval, but she felt she had entrusted her hundred pounds to the right sort of stockbroker' (p. 154). However, the cost of this respectability can be high: a kind of living death. In Maurice's case this feeling is exacerbated, because for him respectability entirely precludes the possibility of human love, the expression of which, because it is gay, would place him outside the cosy circle. Thus, several episodes of dark despair are recorded, and linked to the acceptance of social conformity. Forster wants not merely to blame society for the parlous state of England – in particular, its people's inability to be true to their own emotional needs, and to allow those of others – but to show how the victims' complicity continues it. We each of us lock ourselves into our own cages; the warders are our inner selves as much as the magistrate and the policeman:

> An immense silence, as of death, encircled the young man [Maurice], and as he was going up to town one morning it struck him that he really was dead. What was the use of money-grubbing, eating and playing games? That was all he did or had ever done.
>
> 'Life's a damn poor show,' he exclaimed, crumpling up the *Daily Telegraph.*
>
> The other occupants of the carriage who liked him began to laugh.
>
> 'I'd jump out of the window for twopence.' (p. 125)

(Forster might be surprised to find that eighty years after writing these lines, the symbolic power of this scene of reading the *Daily Telegraph* on a commuter train remains unchanged.) In a particularly fine passage, Forster states his doctrine of struggle; that contending against difficult odds in the teeth of opposition at least offers the possibility of fulfilment, but comfort and security – especially if built on the deprivation of others, and an unseeing complacency – strangle the spirit of love at birth:

> The clientele of Messrs Hill and Hall was drawn from the middle-middle classes, whose highest desire seemed shelter – continuous shelter – not a lair in the darkness to be reached against fear, but shelter everywhere and always, until the existence of earth and sky is forgotten, shelter from poverty and disease and violence and impoliteness; and consequently from joy; God slipped this retribution in. He saw from their faces, as from the faces of his clerks and his partners, that they had never known real joy. Society had catered for them too completely. They had never struggled, and only a struggle twists sentimentality and lust together into love. (p. 202)

In charting the way that the dead hand of uniformity prevents the development of the human heart, Forster is systematic. He begins with the blundering prep-school sex talk of Mr Ducie, with all its shamefacedness about physicality and the concomitant secrecy:

> It is not a thing that your mother can tell you, and you should not mention it to her nor to any lady, and if at your next school boys mention it to you, just shut them up; tell them you know. (p. 7)

The substance of the talk, which is a blend of anatomical diagrams in the sand combined with highminded sententiousness about marriage – 'To love a noble woman, to protect and serve her – this he told the little boy, was the crown of life' (p. 8) – is not dissimilar to the official government line on sex education being advocated in Britain at the time of writing (1991).

At his public school, Maurice is a relative success; that is, without truly distinguishing himself, he imbibes the school's institutionalised bullying (both suffering from this, and practising it against others when he is himself senior) and learns that hardness and insensitivity are required, as proofs of manliness: 'Dr Barry had asked him to befriend a little nephew, who had entered the school that term, but he had done nothing – it was not the thing' (p. 19). At the Prize Day before his leaving, Maurice wins a contest for a Greek oration which is mediocre. The head speaks favourably of Maurice:[2] 'The school clapped not because Maurice was eminent but because he was average. It could celebrate itself in his image' (p. 18). The comforting harmony of middle-class certainties is seductive. Maurice, at this stage, wonders whether it is reality itself ('Was this the world?' – p. 19).

An early uncertainty – structurally matching that at the end of the first chapter, when the fourteen year old Maurice is suddenly overcome by the idea that the respected teacher Mr Dulcie is in fact a coward and a liar, in his sex talk – comes at the Prize Day with his conversation with Dr Barry. The latter is discreet and indirect, but it transpires that he is offended by the immaturity of Maurice's enthusiasm for warfare, in the light of Dr Barry's own recent bereavement: his brother has recently been killed in a war. This disparity, between the fine-sounding official sentiments of a rotten society, and the truths which individuals need to know and live by in order to fulfil themselves morally and emotionally, is to resound throughout this novel. In this particular incident, there is a fine irony in that Dr Barry, who here poses as (at least impliedly) an impatient critic of patriotic flag-waving, re-emerges later in the novel as a medical traditionalist of the worst sort, who tells Maurice that the latter's self-identification as homosexual is simply 'rubbish' (p. 146).

The world of medicine, like that of the public school, represents the official version of the world. In addition to Dr Barry's simple ignorance, we have the casual insouciance of Lasker Jones, the hypnotist. In place of Dr Barry's shocked dismissal, we have in Jones the detached, non-judgmental practitioner. In fact, of course, the very process of attempting to change someone's sexual orientation is, even to the Forster of 1914, deeply suspect, and there is an absurd element to the session in which Maurice steps over a 'crack' in the carpet as he advances towards the imagined picture of Edna May: an absurdity recalling the implied author's distaste for the then-fashionable Freudian theories of the unconscious.

Education, the world of business, and medicine, all conspire against a true emotional development in general, and specifically they thwart and intimidate the gay man as he grows up. To this trinity of the establishment, Forster adds Christianity, which is taken up extensively in the novel through the general discussion of belief, and specifically through the character of Penge's vicar, Mr Borenius.

Maurice falls away from Christian faith at Cambridge under the influence of the atheist Clive. In the case of both men, this lack of faith is seen as positive largely because it is resisted by the families for social reasons rather than doctrinal ones. On one occasion Mrs Hall, seeking to partly excuse Dr Barry's unorthodoxy and contrast it with the doubts of her son, says of the doctor, 'He is a most clever man' (p. 45), meaning to indicate that less clever men (her son) should not have the impertinence to follow the doctor in questioning tradition. This defence of faith is, of course, amusingly flimsy.

Mr Borenius personifies the anti-life spirit of Christianity. The healthy animal spirits and vivacity of the servants are contrasted to his petty alarm over their lack of the sacrament of confirmation: '"But Mrs Durham," he persisted. "I understood so distinctly from you that all your servants had been confirmed."' If only he had been told about Scudder – who is just about to depart for the Argentine – in plenty of time, 'this crisis would not have arisen' (p. 175). This exaggerated fuss over confirmation makes the vicar laughable even in the eyes of the orthodox Mrs Durham. Using a long-standing and, some would say, facile literary device (Dickens's Uriah Heep and Mr Squeers are typical examples), Mr Borenius is rendered additionally offensive by being ugly: 'If the parson hadn't looked so damned ugly he [Maurice] wouldn't have bothered [to answer back], but he couldn't stand that squinny face sneering at youth' (pp. 175–6). In one sense this is laudable: the ugly vicar trying to get his revenge on the young for his own sexual disappointments – the classic Christian mission – gets his come-uppance from Maurice. But, looked at another way, it has the sinister undertone of discriminating in favour of, and overvaluing, the beautiful, *as people,* which we notice in the poems of Cavafy.

Borenius's final appearance, at the port to see Scudder off for South America, features a denunciation of sexual indulgence. In what is clearly a reference to criminal sanctions against gay men, which Forster pessimistically felt throughout his life were unlikely ever to be lifted, the vicar opines that 'until all sexual irregularities and not some of them are penal the Church will never reconquer England' (p. 222). Borenius thinks Scudder has been with a *girl.* We can see here Forster trying indirectly to enlist the support of heterosexuals, by identifying a common enemy in the anti-sex church.

Thus, the mighty institutions of church, medicine, education and polite society all unite to deny basic human needs. But Forster emphasises the collaboration of the victims. Time and again, Maurice identifies his needs and impulses as pathological, and tries through self-restraint, the seeking of medical advice and even the contemplation of suicide, to escape the inescapable. His eventual acceptance of his sexuality, and the consequent cessation of his long, painful journey away from love and desire, are what constitutes the individual victory of Maurice against the world. But the emancipation is expensive; he must leave behind his class, his place in society, his safety, and do battle alone; or almost alone, for he has Alec. *Duo contra mundum*

This depiction of a suffocating Edwardian society is clearly not dated in the sense defined earlier. At the present, the Western world is still in the grip of a homophobia which, in certain cases (notably in Britain) is becomingly more and more vicious. The details and vocabulary differ from Edwardian times, but the root prejudices do not. The Church still denounces gays (or 'pansies' as Dr Runcie, the previous Archbishop of Canterbury, calls us). Medicine and the law still ensure that members of their professions, from judges and hospital consultants to the most junior ranks, remain in the closet or forfeit advancement (and sometimes their current job). Maurice's *Daily Telegraph* still maintains an editorial policy of violent hostility to legal and social equality for gay people, not only in regard to the age of consent for men, but in respect of housing, child adoption, lesbian custody cases, couples' pension rights, media access, employment protection, AIDS/HIV information services, and welfare and counselling rights. All national newspapers support *some* of these anti-equality policies; and most of them, most. In a different way television, through comedy stereotypes and current affairs coverage, marginalises and ridicules the gay experience. British education, from the compulsory Christianity of primary and secondary schools to the distortions of literary criticism in the universities, is still an untaken citadel.

But even if we accept that the novel is powerfully modern in its attack on the institutions of official culture and power, many readers have expressed unease at the development of the plot and certain aspects of characterisation. That is, they have found that a satisfaction with the depiction of Edwardian life in general has to be set against a kind of unsuccess resulting from improbability and melodrama. The idea, for example, that a conservative stockbroker and an undergamekeeper are going to be able to escape into what (with echoes of the outlaw status of Robin Hood) Forster calls 'the greenwood', and live there happily is, at best, implausible. It is possible to argue against this objection that the ending should be seen as metaphorical – Forster's assertion of the power and validity of fighting, with the rewards it must, in the end, bring – rather than probable or realistic.

The objection still remains, however, that in contrast to the mundane world, Forster sets up a series of Arcadias: the greenwood,[3] Ancient Greece (a favourite ploy with gay writers and painters), Cambridge. Hostile critics view this as an escapism – not unconnected with Forster's own life, the beginning and end of which was spent in the Cambridge 'idyll' – and a refusal to address what is, in this argument, called 'the real world'. However, it is now almost universally understood that the Edwardian society of magistrates, priests and stockbrokers (or any other type of society) is no more 'real' than the greenwood or the university enclave. That is, every society, institution and mode of life creates for itself an explanatory mythology which exists to justify and maintain itself. The notion of a 'real' world in this colloquial sense is simply misguided.

I want to conclude this chapter with a more detailed look at the novel's treatment of sex. Although the main thrust of the work concerns homosexuality, we shall see that many of Forster's points are relevant to sexuality generally.

The early hints, in Chapter Two, of Maurice's sexual interest in the garden boy George are subtly done. When Maurice returns home from school, he asks his mother where George is, and is told that he is no longer employed. Maurice's only response is 'Oh' (p. 11). On the next page, he asks the coachman about George, and doesn't appear to have any conscious reaction to this coversation. But during the night sometimes, 'he remembered George. Something stirred in the unfathomable depths of his heart. He whispered, "George, George." Who was George? Nobody . . .' (p. 13).

One sometimes has the feeling that Forster uses the dramatic, symbolic gesture to cover his apparent inability to give satisfactory detailed descriptions of states of feeling. The calling of 'George' is echoed even more symbolically and improbably later in the novel when Maurice leans out of his bedroom window at Penge to pronounce 'Come' in his sleep (a summons answered, of course, by Alec). This inability is more obviously illustrated by Forster's habit of concluding sections, or whole chapters, with sentences purporting to be richly suggestive but actually being meaningless, or at the very least hopelessly unfocused. For example, the above passage about George concludes: 'He did not know that when he yielded to this sorrow he overcame the spectral and fell asleep' (p. 13). The previous chapter (Mr Dulcie's 'talk') ends with: '"Liar, coward, he's told me nothing." . . . Then darkness rolled up again, the darkness that is primeval but not eternal, and yields to its own painful dawn' (p. 9). This could be a sign simply of the artistically crass, giving ammunition to those (F. R. and Q. D. Leavis, for example) who have always claimed second-rate status for Forster. It could also be a sign of that blockage resulting from the author's own repressed feelings. For all his skill, Forster was the product of the inherited sexual guilt of British culture, and speaking openly and directly of feelings of any kind, even through the medium of fiction, would have been difficult. Symbolism is less embarrassing.

Viscount Risley, when introduced, is presented as something of a caricature: 'He made an exaggerated gesture when introduced, and when he spoke, which was continually, he used strong yet unmanly superlatives' (p. 22). The 'unmanly' is a puzzle; so easily it could be Forsterian irony, in which case the meaning would be something like: heterosexuals are so straitjacketed that even verbal exaggeration is taken to reflect on one's virility. But it could easily be taken at face value, with Forster (if we agree to equate him with his narrator, which I think is essential in this novel) sharing the prejudices about what should be considered manly. We hear later that 'in each of his sentences he accented one word violently' (p. 23). The narrative tone is detached, almost scientific. It appears to sit uneasily on the border between mere description and ridicule, and neatly illustrates Forster's ambivalent position about how far to accept society's own norms of what is ridiculous and what is not. I think Forster in his honesty wants to acknowledge the existence of effeminate gay men conforming to the stereotype, but at the same time he is determined that a manly, sports-oriented boxer, Maurice, should in fact stand more fittingly for the situation of gay men. Again, this is all very modern, for 'minority' plays, films and novels are constantly examined for the inner tension they display between providing positive images of minority individuals, and avoiding an improbably good and therefore distorted picture. (Arguments over the representation of gays and Asians in Hanif Kureishi's film, *My Beautiful Launderette* in the 1980s typify this process.)

Forster points out that the effect of oppression on any victim is that it is the victim who feels the guilt, more strongly than the oppressor. This has today become especially well known not only for gay people, but in the case of rape victims. Thus, Maurice feels that 'in all creation there could be no one as vile as himself . . .' (p. 22)

But Forster was himself raised like Maurice, and whatever his intellectual commitment might be, this background makes itself felt in the narrator's remarks:

> As soon as his body developed he became obscene. He supposed some special curse had descended on him, but he could not help it, for even when receiving the Holy Communion filthy thoughts would arise in his mind. The tone of the school was pure – that is to say, just before his arrival there had been a terrific scandal. The black sheep had been expelled, the remainder were drilled hard all day and policed at night, so it was his fortune or misfortune to have little opportunity of exchanging experiences with his school-fellows. He longed for smut, but heard little and contributed less, and his chief indecencies were solitary. Books: the school library was immaculate, but while at his grandfather's he came across an unexpurgated Martial, and stumbled about in it with burning ears. Thoughts: he had a dirty little collection. Acts: he desisted from these after the novelty was over, finding that they brought him more fatigue than pleasure. (p. 16)

The word 'obscene' in the first sentence indicates that Maurice masturbates. This usage, and other key words like 'indecencies' (a legal coinage), 'smut' and 'a dirty little collection' all suggest that, in sharing with his enemy, the establishment, this set of pejorative terms, Forster is less emancipated than he might think himself to be. On the other hand, it is possible that free indirect style (sentiments apparently held by the narrator but actually – the reader has to be sensitive enough to infer this – held only by the character being described at the moment) is being used.

We might interpret what Forster is up to as a dishonest, though in his view no doubt justifiable, ploy. Under this view, Forster begins the novel apparently subscribing to orthodox views of sexuality; then he introduces a pure and platonic love affair between Clive and Maurice at Cambridge – the insistence on chastity here, even to the extent of Clive refusing to kiss Maurice, is heavy – and only having thus laboriously prepared the ground does he introduce the carnal. But even then, he does so only impliedly and with nothing explicit. In other words, the novel is embarrassed by its advocacy of fully fledged (that is, including physical sex) homosexuality.

Maurice has often been found sentimental – but usually by

those who resent being moved by the plight of those whose oppression they would prefer not to have drawn to their attention; and also, of course, by the sophisticated. To me, it combines a strong, successful critique directed against Edwardian hypocrisies (most today firmly in place) with a spirit of defiance which exhilerates even those readers able to see the novel's many flaws.

5

The Love Poetry of the First World War

No one turning from the poetry of the Second World War to that of the First can fail to notice there the unique physical tenderness, the readiness to admire openly the bodily beauty of young men, the unapologetic recognition that men may be in love with each other.

(Paul Fussell)[1]

I can never express in writing what I feel about the men in the trenches; and nobody who has not seen them can ever understand . . .

(Lt-Col. Richard Fielding, in a letter to his wife)[2]

When the war ends I'll be at the crossroads; and I know the path to choose. I must go out into the night alone.

(Siegried Sassoon)[3]

The love of soldier for soldier has always been more controversial than the issue of male homosexuality in general. Two points are, in particular, noteworthy. The first is that the intensity of this love is frequently, perhaps usually, greater than amongst non-combatants, if diaries, letters and poems are to be considered true reflections of writers' states of mind.[4] This is hardly surprising, given that human ties are always more intense during periods of extreme emotional experience (in a mine, a disaster, a shared grief).

It is upon the second point which I wish to dwell. There is, amongst heterosexuals, an especially strong desire to 'exonerate' soldiers (as opposed to men in general) from the imputation of homosexuality. In the 1970s, Field-Marshall Montgomery (he of the North Africa campaign in the Second World War) averred that *there were no homosexuals in the Western Desert.* Although in itself risible, this statement issues from a set of attitudes very widely held and not at all difficult to understand.

Men in general, according to heterosexual opinion, must be seen to conform to certain 'masculine' stereotypes for all the obvious social reasons which the literature of sexual politics has so exhaustively explored in the last twenty years – group solidarity and identity, unity in the domination of women, and so on.[5] But soldiers are not merely individual men; in what they do and how they behave (fiercely, obediently) they are a collective symbol of the controlled virility and power of the society itself. This symbolism is extraordinarily potent, and is attested in scores of observable modes of behaviour. For example, the mere wearing of a military uniform is thought to confer sexual attractiveness and virility on its wearer. In the 1990 Gulf crisis, with Iraq's invasion of Kuwait, on the occasion of the British Government's sending of air force and navy personnel to protect Saudi Arabia, the normally hysterical headlines of the British *Sun* newspaper simply said: 'Our Boys Go In'.[6] Superficially matter of fact, the wording carries a raft of slavishly patriotic and masculist undertones. They are 'our' boys, suggesting both unity of national purpose and a refusal to accept the idea that there might be any dissent from Government action; or if there is dissent, it is marginal and contemptible. They are 'boys', suggesting both the youthfulness and fitness which well equip them for their martial role, but at the same time suggesting their childlike, and therefore moving, vulnerability. (Ironically, 'boys' is favoured both by gay men for its sexual charge, and by straights who use it with a fraternal sense: it is, for example, constantly heard in board meetings and trade union meetings.) Finally, 'go in' is a calculated piece of stiff-upper-lip English understatement. Pride in the unquestioned courage of the forces, it seems to tell us, makes any hyperbole not only unnecessary but distasteful.

I have dwelt on this at some length because it would be difficult to overestimate the resistance amongst heterosexuals to the idea that men *upon whom otherwise they would wish to bestow their deepest admiration,* might have enjoyed other men carnally. Even an ultra-radical in sexual matters, and a scientist and intellectual (of sorts) like the poet Shelley, simply refused to believe that anal penetration and certain other physical expressions of love existed amongst the ancient Greeks:

> We are not exactly aware . . . what the action was by which the Greeks expressed this passion. I am persuaded that it was totally different from the ridiculous and disgusting conceptions which the vulgar have formed on the subject, at least except among the more debased and abandoned of mankind. It is impossible that a lover could usually have subjected the object of his attachment to so detestable a violation or have consented to associate his own remembrance in the beloved mind with images of pain and horror.[7]

The issue goes to the heart of the nature of war poetry itself, and the way in which it was (and continues to be) received. The central question is this: what is meant by saying that one soldier loves another? What did the writers themselves, the addressees of the poems, the readers of the published work, take it to mean? Modern readers find this more of a problem than contemporaneous ones, because of the lifting of the taboo on the discussion of homosexuality. In 1914 it was still acceptable for a man to profess his love for another man, and this was possible partly because the question of sexual deeds did not usually arise as a possible consequence of that profession (whether or not there actually was sexual desire).

A further problem is that different kinds of love are often expressed in the poetry so similarly, that it is by no means easy to distinguish them. Conventions of expression sometimes make brotherly affection, physical tenderness and sexual desire all sound the same. Difficulties of this sort, which arise in any study of 'gay' writing (what is it?, who is included?), are often resolved by a special use of terms: 'homosexual', 'homoerotic', 'gay' and so on, are used in distinguishing ways. Another obvious procedure for me to adopt in this chapter is to confine myself to poets who were certainly (Sassoon) or almost certainly (Owen) gay, and simply write about their work. However, this would drastically inhibit a discussion of very many poems of love, and I have therefore decided instead to adopt an approach suggested by Martin Taylor's anthology *Lads. Love Poetry of the Trenches*.[8] This is, simply, to consider relevant all poems by soldiers expressing their love for other soldiers, whatever kind of love (and it is often a matter of guesswork) it might be.

The result of this approach, as indeed, far more so, of reading the poems themselves, is liberating in a sexual politics' sense, because it underlines the arbitrariness of the 'gay' category. By this I mean that the arrangement whereby certain social and political imperatives require the division of people into categories according to the nature of their sexual desire is historically recent and probably temporary. Just as in the nineteenth century, great importance was attached to dividing people into, for example, Anglican/Non-Conformist, which distinction gradually ceased to have much social meaning, so the division of people into categories of sexual desire would seem also likely to wither. These poems are liberating because reading them assists this withering.

A great many poems explicitly claim same-sex love as superior to men's love for women:

> I found in Hell
> That love of man
> For men – a love more true
> Than women tell
> Since love began.[9]

Commonly, the soldiers' sexual desire for women dries up, because the memory of the 'greater love' makes it appear gross. The speaker in Richard Aldington's single quatrain poem pretends to be asleep to avoid sex:

> Though you desire me I will still feign sleep
> And check my eyes from opening to the day,
> For as I lie, thrilled by your dark gold flesh,
> I think of how the dead, my dead, once lay.[10]

Poets who would not have wanted to sleep with women in the first place often adopted this particular format, as a cover to allow them to express their love without arousing too much 'suspicion'.

> I, that have held strong hands which palter,
> Borne the full weight of limbs that falter,
> Bound live flesh on the surgeon's altar,
> What need have I of woman's hand?
> I, that have felt the dead's embrace;
> I, whose arms were his resting-place;

I, that have kissed a dead man's face;
Ah, but how should you understand?
No I can only turn away.[11]

Equally, poets notorious for their homophobic attitudes and their flaunted heterosexuality, like Robert Graves, echoed the sentiment that men's love for each other was a special thing. In 'Two Fusiliers', the speaker asks what human bond can be so close, and indeed so beautiful, as the soldier's 'wet bond of blood', nurtured by Death.[12]

Studdert Kennedy, a padre during the war and here adopting an ordinary (not 'educated') soldier as his speaker, actually calls his poem 'Passing the Love of Women':

Yes, I've sat in the summer twilight,
Wiv a nice girl, 'and in 'and,
But I've thought even then of the shell 'oles,
Where the boys of the old Bat. stand.
I've turned to 'er lips for 'er kisses,
And I've found them kisses cold,
Stone cold and pale like a twice-told tale,
What has gorn all stale and old.
And the light in 'er eyes 'as gorn all faint,
And the sound of 'er voice grown dim
As I 'eard the machine guns singin' aht,
A-singin' their evenin 'ymn.
Yes, I've known the love ov a woman, lad,
And maybe I shall again,
But I knows a stronger love than theirs,
And that is the love of men.[13]

Later in the poem, the link between enduring pain and the bond of love is made explicit: 'But your comrade Love is stronger love,/'Cause it draws ye back to 'ell.' The speaker in a George Lewis poem tells his loved one, 'You were gentler than a woman when you dressed a wounded limb'.[14] Appropriately enough, the poem is entitled 'To My Mate', consciously or not evoking both senses of the noun.

We notice that many of these poems, reminding us in this respect very much of Whitman's poems about wounds and hospitals from the American Civil War, are gory. The motif of bandaging the bleeding wound of a loved one is found not only in Whitman but also in Hart Crane ('Episode of Hands'). Its popularity is hardly surprising, for a wound renders the sufferer vulnerable and therefore more dear; the wound provides an opportunity for the lover to be solicitous towards the loved one. Some of the poems about injuries can be vivid and gruesome. The near certainty one has that they arise from authentic personal experience saves them from what might otherwise be a charge of tastelessness. In the anonymous 'Dicky Boy An' Me', a shared disaster, and a wounding which anyway puts them out of the running as far as sex is concerned, cements the male bond and renders women supererogatory:

Oh, you can keep your Lizzies and your Nellies and your Sals –
They wouldn't be no good for Dick an' me.
'E's lost 'is leg, I've lost me arm, but we don't give a damn,
'Cos between us we've a proper kit, you see!

And when we wants a smoke o'nights up gets a pair o' legs.
'E's got two 'ands to fill the pipes, you see.
We've got our little pension and we've got our little fire,
An' I've got Dick an' Dicky Boy's got me![15]

There is often an unpleasantly sexist aspect to this. The unwanted women are seen as primarily sexual beings, probably promiscuous, and possibly part of the contingent of armchair warriors urging on the men to fight from the safety of English soil. Owen's character in 'Disabled' signs up 'to please the giddy jilts',[16] and Sassoon is almost hysterical in 'Blighters' as he excoriates the 'prancing ranks/Of harlots' wallowing in the blood-lust of war patriotism.[17]

Both the intensity of male friendships and the marginalisation of women were a consequence of, amongst other things, the public school system from which most of the poets who were published at all widely emerged. Brought up on the twin pillars of Christianity and Imperialism, as embodied in the writings of Kipling and Rider Haggard, they had been imbued with particular values: personal honour, working together, stoicism and a sense of responsibility. The prefectorial system strengthened this code, and the experience of it made possible something quite extraordinary: the more or less direct transition of eighteen-year-old boys into officers at the front. The mere fact that this transition was possible is sufficient to indicate the sort of training and mental and physical preparation which the public schools provided.

E. A. MacIntosh's 'In Memoriam'[18] is a poignant illustration. The poet was twenty when first commissioned as an officer, and twenty-six or twenty-seven when he died. Yet the tone of the speaker of the poem (surely autobiographical), which commemorates one of his privates, David, killed in action, is paternal. The argument, following hints in Ibsen's *The Wild Duck* and anticipating Arthur Miller's *All My Sons*, is that the officer's responsibility for his men is far more onerous, and involves more emotional commitment, than 'mere' fatherhood: 'You were only David's father/But I had fifty sons . . .'. At the end of the poem, he repeats the point, now including all his men: 'For they were only your fathers/But I was your officer.' The emotional charge of the poem resides, of course, in advancing a claim which would in normal circumstances be considered absurd and impertinent: especially as the claims of a parent are traditionally viewed as perhaps the strongest of all.

The idea of 'innocence' was part of the public school ethos; this involved an uncomplicated acceptance by the pupils of the truth and value of the various mythologies (Empire, God, Class and so on) which were offered to them. It explains – what is mostly absent from Second World War poetry – the heroic and pious vocabulary. For example, in First World War poetry (exceptionally, there are some poets like Charles Sorley who avoid this) everyone is 'noble': 'The long, long rest you nobly won';[19] 'But still he died/Nobly . . .'[20] Sassoon, describing a soldier being blown up, tells us: 'So Tommy left us, a gentle soldier, perfect and *without stain* [my italics]. And so he will always remain in my heart, fresh and happy and brave.'[21] (The phrase 'without stain' is used in Catholicism, in Latin (*sine macula*), to describe the Virgin Mary. The word 'stain' occurs again and again in the war poetry.)

Nichols sounds like Henry the Fifth: 'All my Young England fell to-day in fight:/That bird, that wood, was ransomed by our blood!'[22] Part of the innocence is a looking back to childhood as to a protected Arcadia, often with the implication that the post-war world could, given the chance, recreate something of the lost bliss even for adults. E. Hilton Young sites his love poem to his dead friend precisely in this landscape, so that childhood innocence, love, and the pastoral tradition all combine movingly. There is none of the bombast and overblown language of the previous examples. I give the full text:

'Return'

This was the way that, when the war was over,
we were to pass together. You, its lover,
would make me love your land, you said, no less,
its shining levels and their loneliness,
the reedy windings of the silent stream,
your boyhood's playmate, and your childhood's dream.

The war is over now: and we can pass
this way together. Every blade of grass
is you: you are the ripples on the river:
you are the breeze in which they leap and quiver.
I find you in the evening shadows falling
athwart the fen, you in the wildfowl calling:
and all the immanent vision cannot save
my thoughts from wandering to your unknown grave.[23]

In retrospect, some aspects of the poets' innocence horrify us. Rupert Brooke's 'Peace', for example, exults in the opportunity that youth has been given by the war to show what stuff they are made of ('Now, God be thanked Who has matched us with His hour'), and compares young men's entry into war as like 'swimmers into cleanness leaping'. Brooke concludes 'Peace' by arguing that 'mere' physical pain and death, which can, he implies, be transcended, will be the penalties paid by the brave.[24] The connection between cleanness and swimming comes up also in A. P. Herbert[25], and Patrick Macgill also uses 'clean' in 'Red Wine' (the wine/blood metaphor is also common, and suggests the sacred, because of the inevitable evocation of Christ's Last Supper):

Now seven supple lads and clean
Sat down to drink one night,
Sat down to drink at Nouex-les-Mines

And then went off to fight;
And seven supple lads and clean
Are finished with the fight,
But only three at Nouex-les-Mines
Sit down to drink to-night[26]

For all these poets, 'clean' seems to carry a kind of sexual *frisson* suggestive of a tantalising chastity.

The love poetry of this war is specifically personal, by which I mean there is an enormous number of poems not exactly turning away from generalities, but certainly intent upon the commemoration of a specific individual. The titles tell the story: 'To W. D. G., J. C. B., and other young soldiers', 'H. S. G., Ypres, 1916', 'Dicky', 'To R. A.', countless 'In Memoriam' poems, and many 'To my Pal', 'To my Mate' and so on. Ivor Gurney offers 'To His Love' as a title. The importance of this is connected with our relationship, as readers, with texts that come out of experiences of personal horror and anguish. Although it is true that many of the poems lack 'literary' distinction, taking that concept in its narrow and technical sense, it is quite properly felt to be unseemly for readers to complain of such deficiencies, such as they are, aware of the mental and physical conditions under which most of this writing was produced. What might warrant censure under circumstances of composition altogether more relaxed – we find sentimentality, facile ideas, clichés, a disturbing and élitist cult of male beauty, and overblown rhetoric – cannot properly be adduced in connection with this war poetry. It might even be argued that the very 'deficiencies' of the verse – rather like the inchoate and stuttering rage of the interviewee on television who has suffered some injustice – give it a more direct appeal and greater poignancy.

In a way reminiscent of Cavafy, there is a strong tendency for the war poets to attempt to intensify the tragedy of war by stressing the wastage of youth and of beauty, usually both. The words 'boy', 'lad', 'youth' are constantly used, and often homoerotically charged. Sassoon's memorable phrase about the fallen, 'The unreturning army that was youth'[27] finds echoes everywhere: 'Their splendid youth is perished';[28] 'All his splendid youth lies dead'.[29] Even Ezra Pound, whose cynicism is evident,

There died a myriad,
And of the best, among them,
For an old bitch gone in the teeth,
For a botched civilization . . .

manages, in the same poem, an elegiac tone which links the wastage of youth with the wastage of youth's beauty:

Daring as never before, wastage as never before.
Young blood and high blood,
fair cheeks, and fine bodies . . .[30]

The emphasis is almost always on the aborted future: what these young men might have enjoyed and of which they have now been deprived. This is an important point because (apart from the logical nonsense of attributing deprivation in any sense to the dead) it carries the implication that the future, after the war, will return to the Edwardian Arcadian England. It is part of the innocence of these poems, and only rarely does one hear a note of doubt, as for example in the final stanza of Richard Dennys' poem:

Soldier-boy, it's a grim old world
(Deny it, he who can),
Who knows that your life would have happier been,
Had you lived to be a man?[31]

There are in fact a number of 'you're better off dead' poems, but we have to distinguish those, like the above, based on a cynical view of human nature, and those which see youth as a high point, followed inevitably by the decrepitude of old age, to avoid which through death can be seen as advantageous and beautiful.

Those who survive a catastrophe usually feel guilty for having survived, especially if they have been very close to some of those who perished. George Steiner and Enoch Powell have both admitted having this feeling very strongly in regard to the Second World War. (Again, it is as logically absurd as the hideously mutilated survivor who regards himself as more fortunate than his dead friend, because he is at least still alive.

But of course we are dealing with psychological states, not common sense.) The love poems take up this theme:

> You went, old man, before me;
> You died as I knew you, game;
> And 'the wonderful days in store' now
> Could never appear the same.[32]

Here, the death of the friend makes the enjoyment of the future impossible, just as the thought of the dead comrades, as we saw earlier, made heterosexual sex impossible. For Wilfred Gibson also, the future cannot have unalloyed pleasures; they will always be tinged by grief:

> We who are left, how shall we look again
> Happily on the sun, or feel the rain,
> Without remembering how they who went
> Ungrudgingly, and spent
> Their all for us, loved, too, the sun and rain?[33]

Edward Shanks's 'Elegy' describes the love of the speaker for his friend, and speculates feelingly on the manner of the latter's death, and the amount of pain he might have had to endure. Interestingly, he too attributes lesser suffering to himself, though the evidence of the poem is itself a kind of refutation of his attempt to play down the severity of grief:

> And you are dead of wounds and I am scatheless
> Save as my heart has sorrowed for my slain.

Shanks goes on to make a point made in scores of similar poems:

> I might have been with you, I might have seen you
> Reel to the shot with blank and staring eye,
> I might have held you up . . . I might have been you
> And lain instead of you where now you lie.[34]

Going on sick leave made soldiers especially guilty. We should remember that both Owen and Sassoon justified their going back to the war (which they morally detested) after sick leave in Scotland, by telling themselves that they could not abandon 'their' men. Sassoon and MacIntosh both write about how it feels to be safe and comfortable, when the men you love are being killed daily. Sassoon's sleep is disturbed by 'the noiseless dead' who come out of the gloom and gather about his bed and whisper to him: 'Why are you here with all your watches ended?'[35] MacIntosh, who did in fact, like Owen, return to the front and was killed, expressed his predicament in the final stanza of 'From Home'. The use of the phrase 'the heart's desire' indicates the intensity of his need:

> So here I sit in a pleasant room
> By a comfortable fire,
> With every thing that a man could want,
> But not the heart's desire.
> So I sit thinking and dreaming still,
> A dream that won't come true,
> Of you in the German trenches, my friends,
> And I not there with you.[36]

Considerable licence was accorded to war poetry, to allow soldiers to express their love for their fellow combatants; it was good for morale. Some exploited this opportunity to indulge in the kind of sensual detail which would otherwise have been unacceptable. Homoerotic desire when publicly celebrated has always had to have a cover. In the immediate past preceding the war, the common disguise was the setting of a poem (or indeed a photograph) in a classical setting. The Uranian poets (Rex Freston, Scott Moncrieff and Philip Bainbrigge, for example), who celebrated boy love, and were an influence on such as Owen and Sassoon, often used this ploy. Modern covers include buddy detective television series (*Starsky and Hutch* and so on) and, as Norman Mailer has pointed out, spectator sports. (In Britain, public sport, especially football, allows men to kiss other men on the field of play, a display which off the pitch can lead to arrest.)

Wilfred Owen is perhaps the most famous of the war poets to indulge in these sensual details: '[I saw] a last splendour burn the heaven of his cheek'.[37] Usually, beauty is adduced whilst at the same time the expression is under control. That is to say (and this is a criterion that the poets might well have considered consciously), lines like these from W. N. Hodgson could just conceivably have been written by a straight:

I saw you fooling often in the tents
With fair dishevelled hair and laughing lips,
And frolic elf lights in your careless eyes . . .[38]

Geoffrey Faber, on the other hand, holds nothing back in 'The Modern Achilles' (even before we begin, the title uses the classical = gay code, and also chooses someone whose male lover (Patroclus) was famous):

The linked smooth muscles round his form,
The ripe blood blooms in his face;
The dark hair-clusters swarm
About his forehead. Grace
Is his, and strength, and virile loveliness
Of limb, and cool address.[39]

Where, time and again, his contemporaries are coy and suggestive, Faber is delightfully blatant in his lust. Here is the whole of 'Mechanic Repairing a Motor-Cycle':

Something in the look of him makes my pulses snatch.
He crouches on the garage floor beside
The patient engine while I stand and watch.
Black dirt and oil and loose blue clothing hide
What can be hidden. But suddenly streaming wide
The sun's rays enter through the door and catch
His neck and by their alchemy are descried
Grace and glory of youth nowhere to match.
Here is the perfect beauty, not aware
Of its own worth, not asking homage due.
Not like those lads whom sculptor Myron knew,
Whose bodies proudly moved in Grecian air
Bending to conscious play and gleaming bare.
Here's soil and sweat, and youth shines godlike through.[40]

Stepping outside the war context for the moment, this is typical of a certain kind of gay poetry: the semi-voyeuristic speaker; the desired one as rough, tough, working class and dirty (but the beauty shines through); the evocation, directly or otherwise, of ancient Greece; the lack of awareness by the desired that he is the object of admiration; and the strong sense that the speaker is gazing at the unattainable, something ideal which must remain as reverie and can never materialise into anything more 'real'. (We have seen most of these features in the poetry of Cavafy.)

Bathing is, for obvious reasons (athleticism combined with near-nakedness), an attractive subject. (As it is in fiction, with the gay bathing scene in E. M. Forster's *A Room with a View*, later echoed in Iris Murdoch's *The Bell*.) In 'Soldiers Bathing', R. D. Greenway celebrates 'You strong and hairy sergeant/Stretched naked to the skies . . .'.[41] In 'The Bathe' by A. P. Herbert, the swimming becomes a short respite from

> . . . what the morrow brings,
> For that may be the end.
> It may be we shall never swim again,
> Never be clean and comely to the sight,
> May rot untombed and stink with all the slain,
> Come, then, and swim. Come and be clean to-night.[42]

Frank Prewett's 'Voices of Women' combines an appreciation of the dedicatee's beauty with an implied resentment at the woman back home searching for information about him. There is a slight suggestion of the male speaker's (the poet's?) jealous rivalry. Now that the beloved is safely dead, the woman cannot get her hands on him. Here are the final stanzas. The speaker in the first stanza is the woman, and in the second stanza it is the male friend:

> Heard ye my love?
> My love ye must have heard,
> For his voice when he will
> Tinkles like cry of a bird;
> Heard ye my love? –
> – We sang on a Grecian hill.
>
> Behold your love,
> And how shall I forget him,
> His smile, his hair, his song;
> Alas, no maid shall get him
> For all her love,
> Where he sleeps a million strong.[43]

It is, surely, only the middle term in the phrase 'His smile, his hair, his song' which gives us the certainty that sexual love is involved here. A man publicly remembering another's song, and (just about) his smile does not compromise his heterosexual status; hair is another matter.

The daily witness to the contrast between male beauty and the war's hideous mangling of it provides the war poets with another favourite theme. MacIntosh talks of 'the strong limbs broken/And the beautiful men brought low'[44] and in the gruesomely entitled 'Carrion', Harold Monro describes the body thus:

Your head has dropped
Into a furrow. And the lovely curve
Of your strong leg has wasted . . .[45]

The opposite to this is even more common: poets who see a special kind of beauty in the mangled or indeed dead body. 'The dead men are not always carrion', claims Richard Aldington, going into a rapture about the body of a dead English soldier found on the fire-step of a trench:

More beautiful than one can tell,
More subtly coloured than a perfect Goya,
And more austere and lovely in repose
Than Angelo's hand could ever carve in stone.[46]

Herbert Read's poem 'My Company (iii)', given here in full, seems to owe much to the macabre details of Renaissance drama; the love is unapologetically sensual:

A man of mine
  lies on the wire.
It is death to fetch his soulless corpse.

A man of mine
  lies on the wire;
And he will rot
And first his lips
The worms will eat.
It is not thus I would have him kissed,

But with the warm passionate lips
Of his comrade here.[47]

Sassoon shared this sense of the war's despoliation of youthful beauty. He is much more careful than most of the other poets to disguise his sexual desire, but in this extract from the 'Memoirs of an Infantry Officer', the calm diction does not at all mask the emotion:

> As I stepped over one of the Germans an impulse made me lift him up from the miserable ditch. Propped against the bank, his blond face was disfigured, except by mud which I wiped from his eyes and mouth with my coat sleeve. He'd evidently been killed while digging, for his tunic was loosely knotted about his shoulders. He didn't look to be more than eighteen. Hoisting him a little higher, I thought what a gentle face he had, and I remembered that this was the first time I had touched one of our enemies with my hands. Perhaps I had some dim sense of the futility which had put an end to this good-looking youth.[48]

Martin Taylor is severe, and I think rightly, about Sassoon in moments like this: 'His compassion for all soldiers sprang from his vision of their individual beauty.'[49]

Sex and death, eros and thanatos, have always been closely linked. Richard Dennys, in both the title ('Better Far To Pass Away') and the first stanza (here quoted) of this poem, seems to relish the idea of death supervening before age has ravished beauty and destroyed the vibrancy of the young. The words are dripping with sexual suggestiveness:

Better far to pass away
While the limbs are strong and young,
Ere the ending of the day,
Ere Youth's lusty song be sung.
Hot blood pulsing through the veins,
Youth's high hope a burning fire,
Young men needs must break the chains
That hold them from their heart's desire.[50]

Dennys goes on to argue, echoing the Keats of 'Ode to a Nightingale' and the Othello newly arrived in Cyprus,[51] that death would now be a welcome friend. He has, after all, 'known a comrade's constancy,/And felt the grip of friendly hands'.

Some of the poems about death approach necrophilia. Geoffrey Dearmer's 'The Dead Turk' opens: 'Dead, dead, and dumbly chill. He seemed to lie/Carved from the earth, in beauty without stain'.[52] (There's the 'stain' image again.) Charles Carrington's encounter with a dead German is equally chilling:

> He lay as he had fallen, in an attitude of running, struck by three shrapnel bullets in the back. . . . His grey eyes were open, and his mouth showed strong white teeth. I looked on him and loved him.[53]

What, we wonder, did these poets make of *ugly* corpses?

Robert Nichols (the only poet here one wants seriously to apologise for) in this poem combines dishonesty (the 'her' obviously never existed), gruesomeness, sexual grossness ('sudden spasm'), stilted language ('oped'), all rendered in a near-hysterical mode:

> O the fading eyes, the grimed face turned bony,
> Oped mouth gushing, fallen head,
> Lessening pressure of a hand shrunk, clammed, and stony!
> O sudden spasm, release of the dead!
>
> Was there love once? I have forgotten her.
> Was there grief once? grief yet is mine.
> O loved, living, dying, heroic soldier,
> All, all, my joy, my grief, my love, are thine![54]

It is the manner in which the soldiers express their love directly that has left First World War poetry with the dual reputation for being sentimental and at the same time unutterably moving. So we have this:

> Chum o' mine and you're dead, matey,
> And this is the way we part,
> The bullet went through your head, matey,
> But Gawd! it went through my 'eart.[55]

and this:

Oh, Stalk, but I am lonely,
For the old days we knew,
And the bed on the floor at Lesdos
We slept in, I and you.[56]

and this:

He was a man . . . I linger where his cross
Shines white among the shadows, and I know
My very soul is strengthened by my loss.
My comrade still in death – I loved him so.[57]

and this:

There are many kinds of sorrow
In this world of Love and Hate,
But there is no sterner sorrow
Than a soldier's for his mate.[58]

and this:

I don't know if you're living still
Or fallen in the fight;
But in my heart your heart is safe
Till the last night.[59]

When Wilfred Owen said in the preface to his poems, 'Above all I am not concerned with Poetry. . . . The Poetry is in the pity'[60] he was speaking, whether he knew it or not, for the writers quoted above. For the most part, they were not interested in being 'writers', or even in writing 'well'; poetry was one of the very few means by which normally reserved Englishmen could express their deepest feelings. It is to miss the point, as well as to be scandalously insensitive to the circumstances, to complain of technical deficiencies or hackneyed phrasings.

Love's anguish is intensified by the unfairness of the world and the arbitrariness of fate. Sassoon's wonderful valedictory poem to a dying soldier in hospital captures the hopelessness. It ends:

He's young; he hated War; how should he die
When cruel old campaigners win safe through?
But death replied: 'I choose him.' So he went,
And there was silence in the summer night . . .[61]

Owen thought that, to future ages, the poetry of the war would bring consolation. In one sense he was absurdly wrong; for a sustained reading of any First World War anthology of poetry is a scarifying experience which can leave the reader distraught. In another sense, however – and this is its central, exhilarating achievement – it repeatedly attests to the indomitable spirit of love, and the selflessness and courage it inspires, amongst gay and straight alike. J. B. Priestley tells us:

> There are those . . . who found in the war, however much they hated it, the deeper reality we all look for. . . . And almost all these men . . . seemed to feel confused and unhappy as the war receded, as if they were drifting away from reality, as if a world with its guns silent was an uneasy dream.[62]

Edward de Stein put it even more succinctly. For those who have experienced the love of comrades in war, 'What can the world hold afterwards of laughter or tears?'[63]

6

Jean Genet: The Autobiographical Works

Jean Genet (1910–86) was deserted by his mother soon after his birth. He was brought up by peasant foster parents and orphanages, before being sent to Mettray Reformatory at the age of ten. After leaving Mettray, he joined the French Foreign Legion, from which he deserted to follow a career of theft and prostitution across most European cities during the 1930s, punctuated by frequent terms of imprisonment. At Fresnes prison, in France, he wrote his first novel, Our Lady of the Flowers *(the first complete version was discovered and destroyed by the authorities; he calmly wrote the book again) and was sufficiently well known as a writer by 1947 to be the subject of a successful petition to the French President (supported by Jean Cocteau and Jean-Paul Sartre) for Genet's release, despite his having recently been sentenced for theft for the eleventh time in France, and having received a life sentence.*

Our Lady of the Flowers *(1949) was followed by the two autobiographies,* The Thief's Journal *(1949) and* Miracle of the Rose *(1951). Other prose works are* Funeral Rites *(1947) and* Querelle of Brest *(1947). After the war, Genet began writing plays, beginning with* The Maids *(1947), and followed by* Deathwatch *(1954),* The Balcony *(1958),* The Blacks *(1960) and* The Screens *(1963). Increasingly contemptuous of (especially student) radical movements operating within the law, he spent time in the armed camps of, first, the Amercan Black Panthers and later, the Palestinian* fedayeen*; his last book,* Prisoner of Love *(1986), is an account of those experiences.*

This chapter is confined to Genet's autobiographical works, identified in the text as T (*The Thief's Journal*), M (*The Miracle of the Rose*), and P (*Prisoner of Love*).[1] This is partly because of their special relevance to the themes of this book, and partly because they have suffered a certain amount of critical neglect by comparison with the fiction and plays, which have attracted considerable attention. It begins by asserting that Genet's vision of the world is based on ambivalence and unresolved paradoxes. Some explanations are given for this, the most important being the writer's relationship to the Sartrean version of existentialism. Genet's writing is examined in the light of existentialist ideas, and problem areas are identified. These are: the moral repulsiveness of Genet's outlook, the insistence on treachery, and Genet's view of the impossibility of mature love. Discussion of love leads to a study of Genet's depiction of the erotic, and we again see ambivalence: both an ugly and sometimes risible machismo, but also a capacity for tenderness. There then follow discussions of (a) what might be thought to be Genet's reasons lying behind his choice of crime as a way of life, and (b) his aesthetics.

Genet describes how, for a period of three years at the Mettray Reformatory, he would, after shitting, wipe himself with his forefinger, because there was never any paper. He continues:

> I love the Colony for having given me such moments. Idiotic vandals – Danan, Helsey, Londres and others [penal reformers] – have written that penal homes for children should be destroyed. (M, p. 163)

All of Genet's writing is infused with this kind of paradox. He writes admiringly of both tenderness and brutality, of love and hate, of strength and weakness. He despises the weak, yet writes almost lyrically of his subjection by Armand and Stilitano; he despises the 'queers', yet is one. He once said that he was a Black who looked like a White (P, quoted in the Introduction, p. ix)

War is a subject for celebration:

> War was beautiful in the past because in shedding blood it produced glory. It is even more beautiful now because it creates pain, violence and despair. It breeds sobbing widows, who take comfort or weep in the arms of the conquerors. I love the war that devoured my handsomest friends. (M, p. 164)

On another occasion he meets an old beggar-woman in the street just released from prison. He has a sudden fancy that perhaps the woman is his mother (Genet's mother deserted him as a baby): 'I know nothing of her who abandoned me in the cradle, but I hope that it was that old thief who begged at night' (T, pp. 14–15). Immediately afterwards his feelings are reversed, and they become a desire to love: if it were indeed her, 'I would weep with tenderness over those moon-fish eyes, over that round and foolish face!' (T, p. 15). This in turn immediately gives place to a desire 'to slobber over her hair or vomit into her hands.' (T, p. 15).

Even when trying to be most candid, he appears contradictory:

> Never did I try to make of it something other than what it was, I did not try to adorn it, to mask it, but, on the contrary, I wanted to affirm it in its exact sordidness, and the most sordid signs became for me signs of grandeur. (T, p. 13)

His delight in sex takes in both the pleasure and pain of fucking:

> When I bugger . . . [ellipses in original to denote omitted name], as I bend farther forward . . . I see the wincing of his features, but also their radiant anguish. (T, p. 28)

Oxymorons like 'radiant anguish' cram the pages of Genet's work; they are a hallmark of his ambivalence about the world. We hear of 'the miraculous unhappiness of my childhood at the Mettray Reformatory' (T, p. 62), and of 'obscene success' (T, p. 111). Within a few pages we read of 'terrible joy' (T, p. 88), 'anxious joy' (T, p. 89) 'bitter joy' (p. 91). How are we to understand this mass of paradox?

First, Genet has himself told us why he applies laudatory terms to things normally considered odious – in order to 'rehabilitate' them:

> However, if I examine my work, I now perceive in it, patiently pursued, a will to rehabilitate persons, objects and feelings reputedly vile. Naming them with words that usually designate what is noble was perhaps childish and somewhat facile; I was in too much of a hurry.

Thus, he tells us that from the brute facts of his life – from 'hunger, physical humiliation, poverty, fear and degradation' – he has 'drawn reasons for glory' (T, p. 92). Secondly, perhaps Genet's preoccupation with himself as 'the enemy', and with the reader as an adversary (a point repeated frequently by the the use of 'you' to distinguish the reader, and his/her moral scheme, from the author's), leads to a vocabulary which is provocative. Finding himself in a detested, normative society which needs certainty and conventionality, Genet supplies uncertainty (the oxymorons and paradoxes) and an outrageous ethical system. Thirdly, he is perhaps desperately, but yet tenaciously, trying to convince himself. Fourthly, he is terribly confused, and the paradoxes are not to be seen as an intriguing and clever game but an honest avowal of the writer's own uncertainty.

Fifthly, art has its own rationale – we do not expect or desire it to be philosophically accurate or logical. Contradictions and ambiguity are natural to it. This point probably sounds platitudinous to the well read, but the lesson has still to be learned by the majority of commentators. (For example, critics are still offering 'readings' of Shakespeare's *Measure for Measure* in order to attempt to reconcile the contending claims of justice and mercy; whereas the play, wonderfully elevating as it may be in the theatre as a dramatic experience, is, on a conceptual philosophical level, a morass of confusion.) Especially since Modernism (but we can see it even in staid Victorians like Gaskell and Trollope, forever presenting us with unsolvable moral dilemmas), the appeal of the irreconcilable, the writer's desire to offer a kind of creative confusion, has been at odds with intellectual coherence or any kind of regularity. Expecting proper philosophy from literary work is asking for trouble.

However, the most complex explanation can be found in Genet's broadly sharing Sartre's existential outlook. This outlook involves the notion that human existence is properly viewed, not as a predictable entity fixed by certain variables (genes, family, health, race, sex, beauty, social environment, etc.) but something created by each individual through their own personal choices, *ab initio*. Anything which infringes this personal choice is a shackle on freedom. To accept instructions on how to live (from society, law custom, religious precepts, fathers-in-law, or other sources external to oneself) or to see oneself through others' definitions, is a treachery to oneself: Sartre calls it 'bad faith' (*mauvaise foi*). This is a crude synopsis, but the philosophy itself is crude. For example, it seems to believe in a clear demarcation between something I decide to do myself and something which appears to be foisted on me, very largely, by various externals; but it is evident that what I decide to do has been moulded by those externals in the first place. For Sartre, the uniqueness of each personal identity and the emphasis on free choice are central; for many modern philosophers, particularly determinists, neither of these things exists at all.

Genet is an adherent of these principles. I do not mean that he has studied the philosophy in textbooks, but that the reasoning for his actions given in his books corresponds closely (in their drift, if not their style) to the academic views put forward by Sartre. (The philosopher's major work, *Being and Nothingness,* appeared in the same year, 1943, as Genet's first novel, *Our Lady of the Flowers.*) It is unusual for a celebrated philosopher to devote so much of his time to a critical study of a relatively unknown writer,[2] and I believe the reason is not merely the agreement in outlook. Sartre did his existentialism, for the most part, in a library; Genet on the streets. The poor, gay, criminal orphan acts out the drama for which the philosopher, in his study, has written the scenario. This must have been irresistible.

Applying this philosophy – or, perhaps more accurately, acting in preferred ways and much later analysing them according to existential doctrine – Genet can prove he is free by being most perverse, for the most perverse are those who accept no laws and no rules. This is made explicit: 'the greater my guilt in your eyes, the more whole, the more totally assumed, the greater will be my freedom' (T, p. 69). We repeatedly find Genet describing a sad delight in the fact of his social ostracism and isolation. The defiant insistence on freedom is clearly there, but so is a pained bitterness:

> Abandoned by my family, I already felt it was natural to aggravate this condition by a preference for boys, and this preference by theft, and theft by crime . . . I thus resolutely rejected a world which had rejected me. (T, p. 71)

In (rare) passages like this, we glimpse the grievous personal wounds behind the grandiose theories of defiance, and it can sometimes seem that Genet hides his true motives of disaffection (which are resolutely personal and fearful to acknowledge) behind a smokescreen of poetic ideology. I 'suspect' Genet of this partly because I suspect myself.

There are differences between Sartre and Genet; for example, often Genet appears to adopt a fatalistic approach to the future which seems quite contrary to the spirit of existentialist choice. More fundamentally still, Sartre stresses in his work the concept of being 'engagé' (committed), often to some political cause (though it could be any other). It is difficult to reconcile such commitment to the notion of existentialist freedom, and we find Genet incapable of total commitment even to causes he supports. He always feels like an observer, out on the periphery; often he likes that feeling. Thus, of the Palestinian struggle, he says that despite the fact that his whole heart, spirit and body was engaged in the strife, it was 'never my total belief, never the whole of myself'. He looks at the Palestinian revolt 'as if from a window or a box in the theatre, and as if through a pearl-handled lorgnette' (P, p. 90). Even the ideology underpinning the fighters' language has to be taken and used ironically:

> When I use words like 'martyr' I don't adopt the aura of nobility that the Palestinians attribute to them. From a slightly mocking distance, I merely make use of the vocabulary.
>
> (P, p. 92)

The thrill of breaking rules informs these books, but Genet is not a writer of the resistance. Most other literary radicals have alternative moral visions; Genet has none. He is a nihilist. He is not remotely like the person whom we might nowadays describe as a liberal reformer, fighting against heterosexism, inequality, brutal penal institutes and all forms of oppression. On the contrary, in the Christian tradition, he is either indifferent to human suffering or sees it as beneficial to the soul. This religiousness leads him constantly to utilise metaphors of sanctity: his thugs are 'saints', their brutalities 'holy' or 'miraculous', and so on. In obsequious deference to this code, Sartre calls his subject 'Saint Genet'.

Genet's ambivalent attitude to prisons and reformatories stems from the contrast between the humiliations of his own lived experience inside their buildings on the one hand, and the *authenticity* of the institutions themselves on the other. In moments of praise, what strikes Genet is the seriousness, the absence of the ersatz, in prison buildings:

> Prison offers the same sense of security to the convict as does a royal palace to a king's guest. They are the two buildings constructed with the most faith, those which give the greatest certainty of being what they are. . . . The masonry, the materials, the proportions and the architecture are in harmony with a moral unity which makes these dwellings indestructible so long as the social form of which they are the symbol endures. The prison surrounds me with a perfect guarantee. I am sure that it was constructed for me. . . . (T, p. 71)

The important function of the system for Genet is that it recognises and accepts. To the despised poor orphan, having a place, being granted a number, a cell, the respect arising out of fear or contempt – all this is better than being ignored. His identity is made real through the enormous and elaborate state rigmarole which is the penal system. It gives him a place. For similar reasons, Genet regrets the abolition of the notoriously brutal overseas penal colonies, as he was also to regret the closing of the Mettray Reformatory as a result of pressure from French penal reformers. Real abjection gives certainty, definition, recognition to the criminal – above all, it is a kind of tribute because it impliedly says: you are so dangerous, so significant, so in need of attention being paid to you, that these extreme and brutal and expensive methods are necessary to contain you. The home prisons are not extreme enough for Genet: 'I am castrated, I am shorn of my infamy' (T, p. 6). On the other hand, 'the slow and solemn agony of the penal colony was a more perfect blossoming of abjection' (T, p. 7).

These prison passages are, in some senses at least, contrary to the existentialist system impliedly advocated elsewhere, for in them Genet seems to wait passively for recognition, which involves considerable deference to others' importance. However, they could also be seen as parallels to himself in their 'good faith': these institutions, like Genet, offer no pretence, stand on their own, exist in their own right.

There is little evidence in the books under discussion of

proselytising the existentialist view. One of their virtues is a sense of take-it-or-leave-it independence, the refusal to recommend that others adopt his ways, and an even more startling refusal to condemn, say, the soldiers, warders and policemen who abuse him and beat him up. We can point to the weakness of this set of attitudes without claiming that Genet consciously advanced it as a tenable intellectual position.

The main weakness is that it is morally repulsive. We see this not merely on an abstract level, but in specific actions of Genet's life. He makes practically no connection between his own experiences of homophobic oppression, and those of other gays, and one of the corollaries of this is that he appears perfectly comfortable robbing and beating up 'queers', who have been lured to some apartment or dark street by the sexual charms of Genet or his partner(s). (To be fair, I have to record that on one occasion, one of his accomplices makes a contemptuous homophobic remark and Genet gives his support to the reply given by another accomplice, that the 'queers' are being robbed because they – the robbers – need money, and any sense of moral superiority or the 'properness' of stealing from the justly despised is out of place and hypocritical.)

He is always telling us about 'faggots' and 'queers' with the very clear implication that he himself has nothing in common with them at all, and without any apparent sense that, for others, he would belong to this group himself. Even today, there exist men sufficiently lacking in personal awareness to be able to say, 'I'm not really gay, I just like sleeping with men'. Perhaps Genet is reserving these offensive words for the outwardly effeminate, or for those who have established a corporate identity (such as the 'Carolinas' of Barcelona, whom he describes) and flourish in groups, as opposed to Genet's own enviously guarded solitude. Perhaps he is employing them, aware of all the ironies to which I have referred, in a contemptous and bored attitude to precisely the sort of questions which I have here adduced. We find evidence for this propensity in his comments on the use of the word 'martyr' cited above.

At any rate, the extent of Genet's self-oppression, and his having internalized the homophobic values of the surrounding culture, can hardly be doubted. What he says here about Bulkaen is true of himself: Bulkaen, who spurned the 'fags', was himself a 'cocksucker':

> When you saw him, with his usual scowl of disgust, spit the words 'little fag' at a jerk, you would never have thought that he himself was a chicken. Thus, there do exist fellows who voluntarily, and out of choice, are, in their heart of hearts, what is expressed by the most scurrilous insult, which they use to humiliate their opponent. (M, p. 123)

Again, 'Divers had brought off, better than I, the wonderful trick of passing for a tough, whereas he had the soul of a fag' (M, p. 46). This is one of only two references in all three books (as far as I can see) in which Genet suggests some acceptance of his identity as a gay man amongst others. Here is the other: 'I had always needed that steel penis [the burglar's 'jimmy'] in order to free myself completely from my faggotry' (T, p. 26)

Genet revels in heartlessness, in being tough; he cannot afford to be weak: 'Though it is a pleasure for me to strut before [the poor], I most definitely deplore being unable to do so with more ostentation and insolence' (T, p. 73). 'Meanness', he admits, is the 'core of my nature' and goes on to explain why:

> When I was poor, I was mean because I was envious of the wealth of others, and that unkindly feeling destroyed me, consumed me. I wanted to become rich in order to be kind, so as to feel the gentleness, the restfulness that kindness accords (rich and kind, not in order to give, but so that my nature, being kind, would be pacified). I stole in order to be kind. (M, p. 61)

In all the work, Genet is uneasy placing himself: is he tough enough, is he criminal enough, is he independent, is he a 'fag'? The ambivalence is repeatedly evident. Take this description of the Carolinas (the effeminate gay men of Barcelona), who form a procession to mourn the passing of an ancient but beloved pissoir (destroyed by rioters in 1933):

> [They], in shawls, mantillas, silk dresses and fitted jackets, went to the site to place a bunch of red roses tied together with a crepe veil. . . . I saw them going by. I accompanied them for a distance. I knew that my place was in their midst, not because I was one of them, but because their shrill voices, their cries, their extravagent gestures seemed to me to have no other aim than to

> try to pierce the shell of the world's contempt. The Carolinas were great. They were the Daughters of Shame. (T, pp. 52–3)

The Carolinas are 'great' but he is not 'one of them'; in a nutshell we see here all of Genet's uncertainty.

Of course, Genet is aware (consciously or unconsciously) that rejecting establishment values in no sense guarantees freedom for the individual concerned: punks, peace protesters, militant humanists, criminals and many others create alternative cultures. They may well be superior to the mainstream, but they are no more free in the existentialist sense, for their rules and customs are just as binding as those of mainstream culture. How can Genet avoid *any allegiance at all?*

The answer – which he gives time and again – is through treachery. If you betray your most cherished ideas, or your closest friends, there cannot be better proof that nothing ties you down, there is nothing that it is inconceivable that you will do. If you believe in nothing, you can do anything. Thus, Genet has sex with a customs officer and immediately afterwards steals his cape and runs off: it is an early episode connected with the need for betrayal, producing the sensation of 'insidious confusion' (T, p. 24) in Genet's mind. At another stage, he is wondering whether to join the French Gestapo during the Second World War:

> The reason I tore out and saved the scrap of newspaper with their photographs [of members of the French Gestapo] was the desire to draw from it food for argument in favour of treason, which I have always endowed with a radiant visage. (T, p. 124)

Again, he admires Stilitano because he recognises him as a bully who is actually cowardly underneath, and when Stilitano squeals on Pépé, Genet dares not reproach him; he is even perhaps 'excited' (T, p. 65) by the treachery. The appeal is, amongst other things, sexual: 'the temptation to betray [is] something desirable, comparable perhaps to erotic exaltation' (P, p. 59).

Genet steals from friends to prove to himself that he has no moral allegiances. For him, treachery is audacious freedom of action: 'They [those who are treacherous] are the only ones I believe capable of all kinds of boldness' (T, p. 68). He tries repeatedly to get to Tangiers, for it is the home of traitors. He carries with him 'still' [i.e. at the time of writing] (T, p. 59) a photograph of the traitor Marc Aubert. There is something strongly abstract about this obsession with treachery. He is attracted to the idea of being a spy, not for the profit or even the danger, but 'Only the idea of treason' (T, p. 39). When travelling companions, or even lovers, desert him without reason or warning, he never complains. He bears the terrible wounds stoically. It is their right, as it is his, should he choose to exercise it, to betray and desert. Much of the charm is in the solitariness, which for Genet is a form of freedom:

> It is perhaps their moral solitude – to which I aspire – which makes me admire traitors and love them – this taste for solitude being the sign of my pride, and pride the manifestation of my strength. . . . For I shall have broken the stoutest of bonds, the bonds of love. And I so need love from which to draw vigour enough to destroy it! (T, p. 36)

Here is a further development. Treachery not merely fits with the existentialist viewpoint, it is the only antidote to one of the forces, love, to which Genet finds himself, often humiliatingly, subservient. He will not accept those chains. He will, in a manner, kill the thing he loves. (See his novel *Querelle*, where this literally occurs.) This freezes the delightful present in the perpetuity of memory, gives it a ghastly perfection, but most importantly, breaks the stranglehold on freedom. Genet tells us succinctly: 'betraying means breaking the laws of love' (T, p. 123).

This is the terrible price for the existentialist Genet: the impossibility of love. There can be sex, prostitution, temporary tenderness, and prolonged unfulfilled desire (for Stilitano, for example) but the acceptance of responsibilities for another, the notion of reciprocity, is rejected. Repeatedly, Genet smashes any relationship which appears to threaten to become love in a fuller and more mature sense. We see this when he charts his feelings for Michaelis. Genet has in the past appeared impressive to his friend, but now that they are both in jail together at Katowice, and both are carrying buckets of excrement from the guardroom, Genet feels debased and is unable to retain his delight in his friend:

> I hated him for being the witness of my downfall after having seen what a Liberator I could be. My suit had faded; I was dirty, unshaved; my hair was unkempt; I was getting ugly and taking on again the hoodlum look that Michaelis didn't like . . . I no longer loved my friend. Quite the contrary, this love . . . was followed by a kind of unhealthy, impure hatred because it [i.e. the hatred] still contained a few shreds of tenderness. (T, p. 80)

The consequent hardness is not surprising: 'His well-meaningness toward me irritated me' (T, p. 80). And so Genet finds a convenient excuse to abuse his friend.

Genet's delight in his friend is thus seen to have been based on power, on being impressive, on the tough image. For someone purporting all the time to reject the conventions of his time, Genet has a preoccupation with dress and deportment which represents more or less the same fatuity as any fashion-conscious chic set. We need to remember how strongly conformist, intolerant and nasty Genet often is. Thus, he 'hated' Charlot because in a moment of weakness he made *with his own hands* a black satin dress so that his girl could cruise for trade. Genet continues:

> In fact, my nerves couldn't stand the provocations, however slight, of a jerk or weakling. I would let my fists fly at the merest trifle. . . . At Mettray I beat the daylights out of a little jerk who ran his hands over the window-panes with a squeaking sound. (M, p. 33)

Always, when Genet is loved, it is intolerable. He cannot bear it, he must smash it up. Salvator loves him to distraction; thus Genet must break with him. He must show Salvator that he, Genet, is so offensive and mean that the latter will, he hopes, experience no regret at the rupture. Genet tells him bluntly that he is going off with another man, ending his remarks with the insult 'fruit' (T, p. 32).

Emotional masochism is at the heart of Genet's relationships. There is self-abasement, with a concomitant misanthropy. This misanthropy can express itself as racism: 'I would have liked to offer myself to the most bestial of negroes . . .' (T, p. 53), or as misogyny: women are associated with 'slightly nauseating whiffs from the open mouth . . .' (M, p. 187). He relishes being of the fraternity of criminals because of their doomed, victim, status. They are more glorious because of their stupidity:

> We know that their adventures are childish. They themselves are fools. They are ready to kill or be killed over a card-game in which an opponent – or they themselves – was cheating. Yet, thanks to such fellows, tragedies are possible. (T, p. 11)

The denial of love forces Genet into novel modes of thought about his feelings, and consequently a novelty of language. Startling thoughts produce startling language, which is sometimes ridiculous, such as the following lyrical flight of fancy about Stilitano's prick. Genet's hand trembles as he does up the waistband of the one-handed Stilitano's trousers, but the bulging treasure within is not to be touched:

> It is not without reason that in India sacred persons and objects are said to be Untouchable. . . . Behind Stilitano's fly was the sacred Black Stone to which Heliogabulus offered up his imperial wealth. (T, pp. 33–4)

The coldness includes an unpleasant amount of tactical calculation, so that Genet becomes like the heroine of a Restoration drama denying her lover access in order to inflame him the more. His tactics are often as labyrinthine as they are ugly; but the usual components are dishonesty and fantasy. Thus, when Genet meets Bulkaen, another prisoner, we note two things: first, he affects indifference; second, he returns to his cell to fantasise about his new love and the ideal future with him, a future which, however, always ends violently in 'murder, hanging or beheading' (M, p. 24).

Remembering his cruel, institutional background at Mettray, it is not surprising that love should have been pre-empted, and the appeal of machismo and authoritarian violence become so strong, so that we find Genet talk of 'my desire for all the manly types: the soldier, the sailor, the adventurer, the thief, the criminal' (T, p. 33). Nor is it surprising that he dreams of the police of Katowice, being especially drawn to those who are brutal or ruthless:

> No sooner was I locked up in my cell than I dreamed of their

> potency, of their friendship, of a possible complicity between them and me, in which, by a mutual exchange of virtues, they revealed themselves, they as hoodlums and I as traitor.
>
> (T, p. 80)

Rarely, there are passages of extraordinary lyrical tenderness. Of Lucien he writes:

> So long as he is not sleeping, I feel the quivering of his eyelids and upturned lashes against the very sensitive skin of my neck. If he feels a tickling in his nostrils, his laziness and drowsiness keep him from lifting his hand, so that in order to scratch himself he rubs his nose against my beard, thus giving me delicate little taps with his head, like a young calf sucking its mother. He is then completely vulnerable. A cross look or harsh word from me would wound him or, without a trace, would cut through a substance that has become very tender, almost soft, elastic. It sometimes happens that a wave of tenderness, rising up from my heart without my even anticipating it, passes into my arms which hug him tighter, and he, without moving his head, presses his lips against the part of my face or body with which they are in contact. This is the automatic response to the sudden pressure of my arm. The wave of tenderness is always met by this simple peck, in which I feel, blossoming on the surface of my skin, the sweetness of a simple and candid boy. By this sign I recognize his docility to the injunctions of the heart, the submission of his body to my mind. (T, pp. 120–1)

Genet's honesty about his own baseness is accompanied by a pride, a conviction that at least in one way he is superior to 'us' (one is reminded strongly of Tolstoy writing repeatedly in his diary of his conviction that he is mightily superior to the rest of mankind):

> You who regard me with contempt are made up of nothing else but a succession of similar woes, but you will never be aware of this and thus will never possess pride, in other words, the knowledge of a force that enables you to stand up to misery . . .
>
> (T, p. 92)

Of his reasons for turning to crime (other than those already considered, based on existentialist ideas) Genet says there were some simple reasons, such as hunger, but: 'revolt, bitterness, anger or any similar sentiment never entered into my choice' (T, p. 8). Are we to believe this? Is this an example of someone too proud to admit he's been hurt – hurt so badly that he can hardly bear to talk about the issue except in supposed jocularity or other forms of indirectness?

We frequently find evidence contradicting his claim. For example, the reason he gives for not wishing to steal in Nazi Germany is clearly based on rebelliousness. He tells us that, normally, crime is anti-establishment and a radical act. However, in a country which has institutionalised crime, in which those in political control are in effect themselves master criminals, theft becomes conventional:

> If I steal here, I perform no singular deed that might fulfil me. I obey the customary order; I do not destroy it. I am not committing evil. I am not upsetting anything. The outrageousness is impossible. I'm stealing in the void. (T, p. 102)

The sexual element of his life of crime (which for him is usually theft, although he also tells of his peddling opium and many juvenile assaults) is strong. Here, for example, he speaks of the jimmy or 'pen' used in burglaries:

> All burglars will understand the dignity that arrayed me when I held my jimmy, my 'pen'. From its weight, material, and shape, and from its function too, emanated an authority that made me a man. I had always needed that steel penis in order to free myself completely from my faggotry, from my humble attitudes, and to attain the clear simplicity of manliness. I am no longer surprised at the arrogant ways of younsters who have used the pen, even if only once. You may shrug your shoulders and mutter that they're scum. Nothing will prevent them from retaining the jimmy's virtue, which gives, in every circumstance, a sometimes astounding hardness to their youthful softness.
> (M, p. 26)

Burglary is a masculine act, done predominantly by males. It involves breaking in; it is tough and audacious. In these senses, it corresponds to a whole set of conventional notions about sexual behaviour, of how straight men must take the initiative and be tough with (ultimately) pliant women. Genet burgles as a way of 'freeing' himself from that 'faggotry' which he himself, having internalised society's values, sees as unmasculine. The thief is one of the 'manly' types (T, p. 33) and as long as Genet steals he has a good chance of evading the 'queer' insult.

The penis/jimmy analogy is pursued even further, into a fantasy of violence:

> I felt in my trousers, against my thigh, the icy jimmy. I amiably wished that a tenant would appear so that I could use the strength that was hardening me. My right hand closed on the jimmy: 'If a woman comes along, I'll lay her out with my pendulum.' (M, p. 29)

Throughout Genet's work, the metaphors of the eroticism of crime are not merely figures of speech, but suggest resonant and palpable physical experiences.

Sometimes the imagery of crime is softer and more palatable. Criminals are 'fraught with crimes as with glamorous insignia' (M, p. 187). In the case of the beautiful, proud murderer Harcamone, Genet's words are usually hagiographic. We are told that Harcamone's crimes 'gave off a fragrance of roses' (M, p. 42) and along with many other criminals, he is repeatedly described in saintly or religious language, a practice which stresses the writer's determination to make crime (indeed, evil itself) holy, and to turn received notions of the glorious on their heads. Ultimately, Genet woos crime: 'With fanatical care . . . I prepared for my adventure as one arranges a couch or a room for love; I was *hot* for crime.' (T, p. 8).

Genet presents the attractions of crime – and, not wishing to allow us to miss their significance, does so in the opening passage of the book – with the lyrical power closely reminiscent of the sweet and tantalising decadence of the corrupt in Wilde's *Dorian Gray*:

> Though they may not always be handsome, men doomed to evil possess the manly virtues. Of their own volition, or owing to an accident which has been chosen for them, they plunge lucidly and without complaint into a reproachful, ignominious element,

> like that into which love, if it is profound, hurls human beings. Erotic play discloses a nameless world which is revealed by the nocturnal language of lovers. Such language is not written down. It is whispered into the ear at night in a hoarse voice. At dawn it is forgotten. Repudiating the virtues of your world, criminals hopelessly agree to organise a forbidden universe. They agree to live in it. The air there is nauseating: they can breathe it. . . . It was because the world contains these erotic conditions that I was bent on evil. My adventure, never governed by rebellion or a feeling of injustice, will be merely one long mating, burdened and complicated by a heavy and strange erotic ceremonial. (T, pp. 5–6)

If we dismiss the fashionable adulation which turns aside from Genet's malignity (Edmund White says that none of Genet's crimes 'amounted to anything more serious than running away from school, boarding a train without a ticket or stealing a book' (Introduction to P, p. ix); a reading of the books would have shown White the drug deals and the assaults) and insist on placing this in the reckoning, it is not in order to be censorious, but to discover, as we need to do if we are gradually to piece together our silenced culture and experience as gay people, exactly what price we have had to pay to homophobic society; for at the end of the day, Genet's books tell us: *this is what they can do to us, this is the extent of their influence.* The cruelty of those who have themselves been cruelly treated is tragically predictable.

I wish now to turn to Genet's attitude to his writing, considered as an art and as an activity:

> For I tear my words from the depths of my being, from a region to which irony has no access, and these words, which are charged with all the buried desires I carry within me and which express them on paper as I write, will re-create the loathsome and cherished world from which I tried to free myself.
>
> (M, p. 33).

Some of the characteristics of Genet's work, which we have already noted, can be seen here. The first phrase tells us of the birth pangs of his writing. There is clearly a contrast between the source of his work, the 'region to which irony has no access', which I take to refer to a kind of exposed rawness painful to contemplate, and the heavily ironic and disguised finished products of the artistic process. This might sound odd in that the books often seem obviously frank. But alongside the apparent frankness, as I have tried to show in the discussion of love and sexuality, there is evasion, lack of clarity, a fear or reluctance to engage in honest self-inspection. Some argue that even the apparently frank passages are an elaborate blind, leading us away from the real raw nerves of Genet's heart. Deception in the guise of seeming disclosure.

The passage once again illustrates Genet's ambivalence ('loathsome and cherished world') towards experience; and the final phrase makes it plain that Genet sees writing as therapy, as his individual way of organising, and thereby making sense of, the world. Where the experiences have been extreme, one can think of this process as a kind of exorcism.

Ultimately, the writing is for him, not us: 'I was as interested in my own curiosity as in its objects' (P, p. 91). This partly explains its difficulty; like Gerard Manley Hopkins, he need make no concessions to intelligibility because his primary aim is not communication with others but communing with himself.

As a modernist, he is aware of the problematic status of prose, and he raises the issue of its purported ability to mirror the world of reality. Throughout the three books, he calls our attention to these issues, telling us not to confuse his account of the past with the 'truth' about that past. He says a true history of the past is impossible: 'our language is incapable of recalling even the pale reflection of those bygone foreign states'. The book 'is meant to indicate what I am today, as I write it. It is not a quest of time gone by, but a work of art whose pretext-subject is my former life. It will be a present fixed with the help of the past, and not vice versa' (T, p. 58). In the final book, the point is laboured:

> The page that was blank to begin with is now crossed from top to bottom with tiny black characters – letters, words, commas, exclamation marks – and it's because of them the page is said to be legible. But a kind of uneasiness, a feeling close to nausea, an irresolution that stays my hand – these make me wonder: do these black marks add up to reality? (P, p. 3)

Again, writing is a process 'leaving on the page nothing but error' (P, p. 27), and, 'Are these pages only a barricade to hide the void . . . ?' (P, p. 74) He concludes that perhaps the materials on which one writes possess more reality than the signs written.

If they were novels, they would be described as having unreliable narrators. Genet frequently makes assumptions and gives us the grounds for those assumptions, and often the latter are ridiculously thin; for example: 'The gentleness of that moon-fish face revealed to me at once that the old woman had just come out of prison' (T, p. 14). This too (intentionally or not) raises the question of what we can 'really' know.

Genet's inadequacies in transcription, in the attempt to set down the essence of his life experience, are part of the attraction of the work. Like Baldwin, the frequent lapses into hypocrisy, even stupidity, indicate a writer unconcerned with the high polish, the faultless artistry, of a Proust. There is a reckless courage in this. He risks a great deal, so that for example certain levels of abstraction or metaphorical reverie just do not work, and seem pretentious: Harcamone's murder is like a poem:

> The author of a beautiful poem is always dead. The Mettray colonists realized this, and we spoke of Harcamone, who had killed a nine-year-old girl, only in the past tense. (M, p. 156)

> This book, *The Thief's Journal*, pursuit of the Impossible Nothingness. (T, p. 77)

As a young prisoner, Genet managed to get hold of a copy of part of Marcel Proust's *Remembrance of Things Past*, and his own writing is massively in the debt of the earlier author. The main borrowings are: first, the belief that when past experience is renewed through memory and captured through the intricate rearrangements and patternings of literary art, the result may well be as infused with life as the experiences which gave rise to it, if not more so; second, an abandoning of the doctrine of the centrality of didactic morality in literature; third, a lyrically rapturous style, a leisureliness of pace, a profound reflection, articulated in an immensely complex syntactical structure, and suggesting self-absorption and reverie, and making considerable demands on readers. Those who know Proust's work will recognise its affinity to passages such as this one about Harcamone:

> And I am going to speak of his death sentence. I shall explain later the miracle whereby I witnessed, at certain times, his entire inner, secret and spectacular life, but here and now I offer my thanks for this to the God we serve, who rewards us by the attentions that God reserves for his saints. It is saintliness too that I am returning to seek in the unfolding of this adventure. I really must go in quest of a God who is mine, for as I looked at pictures of the penal colony my heart suddenly clouded with nostalgia for a land which I knew elsewhere than in Guiana, elsewhere than on maps and in books, and which I discovered within myself. (M, p. 400)

Proust, along with the English aesthetes, is able to dislodge the morally didactic from the centre of literature because he can put in its place something else: the idea of life itself as art and as spectacle. This is a point of view which requires detachment and is frequently to be found in gay writers, who have it by virtue of their social ostracism.

Genet also sees life as spectacle and theatre and what he has to say about the Black Panthers is of crucial importance here, as it is fundamentally an explanation of his own life:

> The Whites recoil from the Panthers' weapons, their leather jackets, their revolutionary hair-dos, their words and even their gentle but menacing tone – that was just what the Panthers wanted. They deliberately set out to create a dramatic image. The image was a theatre both for enacting a tragedy and for stamping it out – a bitter tragedy about themselves, a bitter tragedy for the Whites. They aimed to project their image in the press and on the screen until the Whites were haunted by it.
> (P, p. 83)

Again, 'the Panthers would do their best to terrorize the masters by the only means available to them. Spectacle' (P, p. 85). Like Byron and Wilde, Genet's attitude to his own life as represented in the autobiographical works is largely informed by the idea of spectacle – from the basic props (a tube of Vaseline taken from his pocket after arrest and lying on the police station table like a terrible reproach which nevertheless fills him with pride; the burglar's phallic 'jimmy') to the whole tragic setting of crime and punishment.

Genet's aestheticism (if we take this to mean the writer's diverting attention away from an expected concentration on the moral and political significance of the events described and offering instead the spectacle of lives as beautiful or theatrical; or, at any rate, as aesthetic objects) has evinced two distinct and contrary responses. The first, from Sartre, in *Saint Genet. Actor and Martyr*, referred to above, is offered as a celebration of Genet's moral courage. Sartre is immensely impressed by Genet for reasons I have fully adduced already. We can summarise them by saying that Genet's disgust of conventional society and the consequent active breaking of its most sacred rules, in acts of crime and forbidden sexuality, is a kind of courageous living display of the existentialist principles which Sartre advocated. In praising his subject for deliberately and unapologetically soiling himself with, amongst other things, the 'perversion' of same-sex activities, Sartre has to accept (and we see it in his own fictional work, such as *Les Chemins de la Liberté* and *Huis Clos*) all the most reactionary assumptions about sexuality. Put simply, homosexuality is only daring if it is assumed to be always disgusting.

A more conventional view appears in *Genet. Dandy of the Lower Depths* by Larry Nachman. Nachman's view is that, in aestheticism as defined above and as specifically represented by Genet's life, one chooses homosexuality because 'to be in an equivocal relation to the ordinary world of one's fellows' may be 'an important and perhaps necessary pathway to a heightened aesthetic and intellectual sensibility'.[3] He compares Genet to Rilke, who refused to undergo psychoanalysis because he thought that being reduced to 'normality' would ruin his talent. This comparison overlooks the different kinds of choice involved in 'choosing' psychoanalysis and 'choosing' homosexuality. (In Genet's work, most of the emphasis is on the idea that his sexual orientation was a 'given', like being an orphan, but which, in one sense, he can still 'choose' in the sense that he does not deny his nature but lives in 'good faith'.)

Nachman then offers a comparison with Proust: the latter makes of his outcast status a kind of refinement; Genet, on the other hand, makes erotic capital out of being spurned. Crime and murder are sexy. And it is sex – promiscuous, impersonal, selfish sex – which Nachman hones in on. Genet treats other men as mere bodies, as fantasy sex objects. He is incapable of 'love' – or, at least, resists trying it out – because he must retain his complete isolation. Occasionally, the burden of this isolation becomes so oppressive that he desires to join with others in 'his desire for revenge upon the world'. Genet is essentially a Nazi: 'He would have been at home in the SA which was, among other things, a cult of decadent homosexual toughs and aesthetes' (p. 369.)

Nachman's analysis comes out of an unapologetic heterosexism; Sartre's out of an idealistic philosophical belief in free choice as the ultimate good, regardless (almost) of the choices involved. Nevertheless, Nackman comes closer to the truth. Genet's view of, and behaviour in, the world, is grotesque, because it is entirely egotistical. If any set of books refuted Wilde's dictum that there are no such things as morally good or bad books, only well or badly written ones, these are they. Their astonishing lyrical power does not disguise the poison they contain.

7

The Plays of Tennessee Williams

Tennessee Williams (1911–83) was born in Columbus, Missouri. At the age of twelve his father, a travelling salesman, moved the family to St Louis, but both he and his sister (with whom he had a close relationship, which is reflected in some of the plays) found urban life unsettling. He spent two years in college before taking a clerical job in a shoe company. He stayed there for two years, writing in the evenings. In 1938 he took a course at the University of Iowa, at the same time having a succession of part-time jobs. After receiving a Rockefeller fellowship in 1940, his plays became increasingly well-known and respected (his short stories and novels have received less acclaim). His autobiography, Memoirs, *was published in 1975.*

In the first part of this chapter I shall be looking at gay resonances in two of Williams's most famous plays, *The Glass Menagerie* and *A Streetcar Named Desire*;[1] in the second part, the discussion is widened to include a more general discussion of sexuality in a number of other Williams plays.

In *The Glass Menagerie* Laura's lameness is, on several levels, a metaphor for Williams's view of homosexuality. (We find it also in *Cat on a Hot Tim Roof* and E. M. Forster's *The Longest Journey*.) First, it is seen as a disability which actually restricts sexual fulfilment. The 'gentlemen callers' that Amanda, Laura's mother, repeatedly insists will come visiting, will in fact never come. At high school, she went unnoticed by the boy with whom she was infatuated. Secondly, the restricting nature of the disability, real as that is, is massively increased by the sufferer's obsession with it:

JIM. Now I remember – you always came in late.

LAURA. Yes, it was hard for me, getting upstairs. I had that brace on my leg – it clumped so loud!
JIM. I never heard any clumping.
LAURA [*wincing at the recollection*]. To me it sounded like – thunder!
JIM. Well, well, well, I never even noticed. (p. 294)

That obsession is aggravated by the refusal of Amanda to accept Laura's condition: she pretends to herself and to Laura that suitors will materialise one day; she forbids the use of the word 'cripple'; when Jim calls, she insists on overriding Laura's desire not to come to the table, thus exposing her to the meeting which is to have such devastating results.

Thirdly, the consequence of her disability and the accompanying desire to retire from the world (it is more acute than mere shyness, for she feels physically sick simply attending the business college Amanda has sent her to) is her absorption in the world of the glass menagerie. It is beautiful, fragile, deeply personal, but considered quaint and unhealthy by Jim, who represents the world of 'normality'. His (unexpressed) hostility to the menagerie is symbolised by his attempts to entice her away from it into his own 'normal' world. He takes her through a truncated wooing: he coaxes her to relax, to laugh, to dance, and finally to accept his kiss. In the process, bumping into the table, her favourite piece, the unicorn, breaks and loses its horn, and therefore its individuality.

The unicorn is an emblem of Laura, who in turn symbolises the individual gay person, isolated certainly, but possessing valuable individuality. There is, however, a crucial difference:

JIM. What kind of a thing is this one supposed to be?
LAURA. Haven't you noticed the single horn on its forehead?
JIM. A unicorn, huh?
LAURA. Mmmm-hmmm!
JIM. Unicorns, aren't they extinct in the modern world?
LAURA. I know!
JIM. Poor little fellow, he must feel sort of lonesome.
LAURA [*smiling*]. Well, if he does he doesn't complain about it. He stays on a shelf with some horses that don't have horns and all of them seem to get along nicely together. (p. 301)

In the 'real' world of the Wingfield household, Laura is unhappy and unfulfilled. In the fantasy world of the menagerie, the 'normal' horses have no quarrel with the 'abnormal' unicorn. Laura's reason for imagining this world is to create a society where her disability will not be problematic. Williams has imagined it to create a world where homosexuality will not be problematic.

But Laura's fantasy of the menagerie is not secure, and this is expressed in the play in at least three ways. First, of course, the animals are made of glass and are constantly being disturbed *inadvertently* by the outside world: 'Glass breaks so easily. No matter how careful you are. The traffic jars the shelves and things fall off them' (p. 303). Secondly, there are deliberate or semi-deliberate attacks: Jim's ingratiating himself with her, leading to the dancing which results in the unicorn being broken, is the example here. Thirdly, she is unable to sustain the fantasy unbroken even within herself; for although, in the above extract, she claims the horses and the unicorn 'get along nicely together', she indicates that before the breakage the unicorn must have felt 'freakish' (p. 303). The parallel with Keats' odes here ('To a Nightingale', 'On a Grecian Urn') is exact. The two objects allow a respite – 'Fade far away, dissolve, and quite forget/ . . . The weariness, the fever, and the fret' – but it is tragically and inevitably temporary. Keats's 'fancy cannot cheat so well/As she is fam'd to do' and Laura's make-believe world is equally disappointing and incomplete.

Thus the menagerie represents the possibility we all possess of living in an individual reality other than and hostile to, the reality foisted on us by society; but this individual reality will probably be found to be vulnerable and fragile.

Laura is not alone in creating an alternative world. Amanda and Tom also have their private realms. For Tom it is, in the short term, escaping the grinding tedium of the warehouse for the excitement of the movies. But the movies are also a con-trick offering vicarious, and therefore unreal, gratification:

TOM. . . . All of those glamorous people – having adventures – hogging it all, gobbling the whole thing up! You know what happens? People go to the *movies* instead of *moving*! Hollywood characters are supposed to have all the adventures for everybody in America, while everybody in America sits in a dark room and watches them have them! (p. 282)

In the long term, his planned escape route is to become a merchant seaman. Domestic boredom and stasis is to be replaced by something perhaps equally unsatisfying, the restlessness and lonely wandering that the seaman's life represents (potent in American literature from Melville to O'Neill). The final monologue stresses both the solitude and the compulsive movement:

TOM. . . . I travelled around a great deal. The cities swept about me like dead leaves, leaves that were brightly coloured but torn away from the branches.

I would have stopped, but I was pursued by something. . . . Perhaps I am walking along a street at night, in some strange city, before I have found companions. (p. 313)

The desire for the seaman's life has a clear gay element, in terms of the desire for an all-male community linked by a common endeavour and the especially intense camraderie which is the product of hardship (gay writing, from pornographic magazines to the elaborate linguistic pyrotechnics of Jean Genet's *Querelle*, reflects the naval fantasy).

For Amanda, the private realm is the past of having seventeen gentlemen callers on one day, and rooms full of jonquils, and being courted by well-mannered planters' sons with huge wealth. Her vision of the past is represented as being not only highly coloured and to some extent illusory, but vulgar as well. And there is enormous skill in the way Williams simultaneously conveys the sordidly mercenary and the romantically elegaic:

AMANDA. . . . My callers were gentlemen – all! Among my callers were some of the most prominent young planters of the Mississippi Delta – planters and sons of planters! There was young Champ Laughlin who later became vice-president of the Delta Planters Bank. Hadley Stevenson who was drowned in Moon Lake and left his widow one hundred and fifty thousand in Government bonds. There were the Cutrere brothers, Wesley and Bates. Bates was one of my bright

> particular beaux! He got in a quarrel with that wild Wainwright boy. They shot it out on the floor of Moon Lake Casino. Bates was shot through the stomach. Died in the ambulance on his way to Memphis. His widow was also well provided for, came into eight or ten thousand acres, that's all. (pp. 238–9)

Similarly, her role as a telephone salesperson trying to get subcriptions to the sentimental magazines pedalling cheap dreams (in her patter she speaks of a story thus: 'It has a sophisticated, society background. It's all about the horsey set on Long Island!' – p. 263) parallels the attempts she makes in her own domestic life to 'sell' a sentimentalized version of love, the future, and the past.

Laura's infatuation with Jim seems almost as sturdy at the time of the play's events as during her schooldays. As the final scene (Scene 7) unfolds, Jim's appalling character gradually becomes apparent to the audience, so that one reasonable expectation at this point might be that the play is to deal with Laura's painful disillusionment. The high-school hero shows himself to the doting adorer as having feet of clay. The opposite occurs. Laura doesn't notice. She doesn't notice his bigotry (the German ex-girlfriend is described as a 'kraut-head' – p. 297), his facile belief in materialism ('Think of the fortune made by the guy that invented the first piece of chewing gum' and, of an exhibition, 'Gives you an idea of what the future will be in America, even more wonderful than the present time is!' – p. 292), his vanity (he offers to autograph the programme for her), and his preachy self-righteousness and superior air. Williams encapsulates his disdain in two details: Jim is keen on public speaking and getting in on the future of television, both emblems of the crass and the phoney.

But Laura's blind love screens out these negative traits; she has a unique view of Jim not rendered any the less valid because it is idiosyncratic. Jim's verbal mishearing of the name of Laura's school illness is a parallel symbolic moment:

> LAURA. I was out of school a little while with pleurosis. When I came back you asked me what was the matter. I said I had

> pleurosis – you thought I said Blue Roses. That's what you always called me after that! (p. 294)

Not only is this Jim's equivalent of Laura's 'mistaken' love – for he in his turn through lexical error turns illness into floral beauty – but it creates a beauty which is also an oddity. Like the menagerie unicorn, it is both uncommon and freakish:

> JIM. . . . [Other people are] common as weeds, but – you – well, you're – *Blue Roses!*
> LAURA. But blue is wrong for – roses . . . (p. 304)

We have seen, therefore, that the play addresses the question of what various strategies can be deployed to escape being defeated by conventional life. I should like, therefore, to say something about the way this conventional life is itself depicted.

First, through the character of Amanda, it is associated with restrictive and tedious rules. The highly comic diatribe from Amanda, which opens the play, concerning the need for the thorough mastication of food, is vigorously opposed by Tom: 'I haven't enjoyed one bite of this dinner because of your constant directions on how to eat it' (p. 236). Later, Amanda tells her son that the amount of money he spends on tobacco could be used instead to pay for 'a night-school course in accounting at Washington U! Just think what a wonderful thing that would be for you, Son!' Tom's rebel reply – it rejects the 'sensible' for the dangerous and the subversively unambitious – is a simple: 'I'd rather smoke' (p. 264). Tom's hostility to both injunctions is based on a preference for immediate pleasure over the decorous, the correct, the long-term view.

Secondly, and following from the previous point, Tom's job at the shoe warehouse is the very epitome of mindless slog, to which even those brilliantly promising in their youth (Jim) must be consigned, unless they choose to deviate from the conventional:

> TOM. Listen! You think I'm crazy about the *warehouse?* You think I'm in love with the Continental Shoemakers? You think I want to spend fifty-five *years* down there in that – *celotex interior*! with – *fluorescent – tubes!* Look! I'd rather somebody picked up a crowbar and battered out my brains – than go

> back mornings! I *go!* Every time you come in yelling that God damn *'Rise and shine!' 'Rise and Shine'* I say to myself, 'How *lucky dead* people are! But I get up. I *go!* For sixty-five dollars a month I give up all that I dream of doing and being *ever!* (pp. 251–2)

Jim, it is clear, has been nailed into this coffin until death. He accepts the incarceration willingly, as though unaware, and the character traits described earlier go naturally with the job. On the other hand, Tom's decision to enter the Merchant Navy is of course the refusal of such deadly conventionality. It is not to be cosy (there will be physical rigours and a wandering unsettled life) and the decision is not easily made (it entails 'deserting' the household of which he is the chief financial stay) but it promises the adventure which hitherto he has had to take vicariously in the cinema.

When Amanda sends Laura out of the house to the grocer's in order to speak to Tom privately, she urges Laura to make haste. The consequence is that Laura stumbles on the stairs. Through this episode we are shown that Laura's problems are not merely the result of her own obsession (as for example with the sound of the 'clumping') but come about through the malign agency of her mother. Amanda lectures and harangues both her children, foisting on them everything from health tips to sub-metaphysical homespun wisdom about life itself. She has the Christian's horror of sexuality ('Christian adults don't want it' (p. 260) she remarks about instinct, in an argument with Tom) and stresses the concept of the superiority of humanity over the animals in a passage (p. 260) which is parallel to one by Blanche duBois in *A Streetcar Named Desire*. Williams shows us that family life, and the influence of parents, can be destructive and miserable, and thus subverts the usually unquestioned view about the pre-eminence of this supposedly normative and healthy mode of life.

In the received wisdom of gay politics, intolerance is the result of sexual denial: the bigot cannot accomodate her/his sexual needs, and the ensuing frustration is partially manifested in an envious determination to prevent the sexual pleasure of others. Amanda's denunciation of 'instinct' in *The Glass Menagerie* is clearly pathological. It is seen in her near-hysterical rejection of the works of D. H. Lawrence. It goes hand in hand with an obsessional attention to the (superficially at least) non-sexual bodily functions; prudes, notoriously, concern themselves with 'being regular' in their excremental habits, and talking about it in public. Thus we have the constant nagging of Tom about chewing his food. In *A Streetcar Named Desire,* as with *The Glass Menagerie,* Williams wants to insist on the primacy of sexual desire. He does it in a gay tradition of writing, which is conspicuously more emphatic, if not blatant, than his heterosexual contemporaries. Desire may well be brief and painful – in *Menagerie* Tom speaks of the 'sex that hung in the gloom like a chandelier and flooded the world with brief, deceptive rainbows' (p. 265) – but it is seen as taking precedence in human affairs:

> STELLA. But there are things that happen between a man and a woman in the dark – that sort of make everything else seem – unimportant.
> BLANCHE. What you are talking about is brutal desire – just – Desire! – the name of that rattle-trap street-car that bangs through the Quarter, up one old narrow street and down another . . .
> STELLA. Haven't you ever ridden on that street-car?
> BLANCHE. It brought me here . . . (p. 162)

Sexual desire is also anarchic, it 'knows no laws' in Chaucer's formula. Blanche's desire for young boys gets her thrown out of her schoolteaching post, and this connection between sexuality and social ostracism also speaks to the gay experience. Indeed, her very schizophrenia is the result of aspiring to both respectability and desire, an attempt to live in the world of animal passion and at the same time that of gentleman callers and the courteously well behaved. These two modes clash throughout the play, especially in Blanche's dialogues with Stanley, where heavy sexual suggestiveness is mixed with Blanche's language of high decorousness:

> STANLEY. My clothes're stickin' to me. Do you mind if I make myself comfortable?
> [*He starts to remove his shirt.*]
> BLANCHE. Please, please do.

STANLEY. Be comfortable is my motto.
BLANCHE. It's mine, too. It's hard to stay looking fresh. I haven't washed or even powdered my face and – here you are!
(p. 129)

The duality is especially well-rendered in scene five, in which Blanche, having been carried away by the young man ('a young prince out of the Arabian Nights' – p. 174) and planting a kiss on his lips, she immediately receives the altogether less sensual and more stolid Mitch – who holds for her the promise not of pleasure but of financial security – with affectation and facetiously exaggerated courtesy:

BLANCHE. Look who's coming! My Rosenkavalier! Bow to me first! Now present them.
[*He does so. She curtsies low.*]
Ahhh! Merciiii! (p. 174)

In *The Glass Menagerie* Tom tells us, in his capacity as narrator, that the play is 'dimly lighted' (p. 235) and for Blanche too, the garish light of everyday must be muted by paper lanterns. One reason for this is that made explicit in the play: her wish to deceive Mitch about her age. But we also feel that Blanche, in a more general sense, cannot stand the light, cannot cope with the cruelties of the outer world. A series of images and events reinforces this need for avoidance: the alcoholism, the retreat to the bathroom (strong connotations here of a futile attempt at washing away her past in Laurel), and the phoney gentility of her clothes, her talk, her home (the name 'Belle Rêve' could hardly be plainer). An eloquent testament to the truth of the idea that Blanche embodies, in her paranoia, isolation, attempts at clinging to both respectability and passion, and retreat from the world, many of the emotional states foisted on gay people by a homophobic culture is that, despite her manifest horribleness of character, many gay students whom I have taught find her sympathetic, tend to withhold their condemnation, and are, indeed, even attracted by her doomed status.

Blanche's life is of love gone wrong: from the disastrous marriage with the gay boy whom she effectively betrays, to the final divided self of madness. Stanley, on the other hand, wins out. He is animal vigour without an encumbering culture. (I shall be developing this point shortly.) The terms in which he is described – see the long stage direction, from 'Animal joy in his being is implicit in all his movements and attitudes . . .' (p. 128) – make it plain how far he is a stereotyped homoerotic icon for Williams himself.

Through the characters of both Laura and Blanche, Williams delivers a bleak verdict on the chances of alternative sexuality. Gay desire, which can be seen as the subtext informing the fortunes of both women, may survive fitfully in hugger-mugger, but must ever shun the light of day. Williams's work precedes the idea, the possibility, of coming out of the closet. In fact, it is the closet that he portrays – how dark it is, and yet often warm, offering a reclusive bolt-hole. Some form of hiding is what these plays ultimately come up with. As gay readers of today, we can use these texts to inform ourselves of part of the history of our psychic oppression, but must determinedly turn away from their negative conclusion.

In later plays, when the opportunity provided by a more liberal climate allowed Williams to discuss gayness directly, the presentation of homosexuality continues self-pityingly bleak. For example, in *Vieux Carré*,[2] the decayed rooming house is typical of the claustrophobic rotting hopelessness of William's settings. In the play, the 'writer' has reluctant sex with the older man, and then imagines his dead grandmother surveying the encounter: 'I felt that she neither blamed nor approved the encounter. No. Wait. She . . . seemed to lift one hand very, very slightly before my eyes closed with sleep. An almost invisible gesture of . . . forgiveness? . . . through understanding?' (p. 27). Thirty years on from the successes of the late forties, Williams is still describing gay experience in terms of forgiveness (and therefore, impliedly, of sin). Melancholy is endemic, as indicated by this line (which Orton was to borrow for *The Good and Faithful Servant*): 'What were you crying about? Some particular sorrow or . . . for the human condition.?' (p. 18).

In *Small Craft Warnings*,[3] we find the following speech given by Leona:

> I know the gay scene and I know the language of it and I know how full it is of sickness and sadness; it's so full of sadness and sickness, I could almost be glad that my little brother died

> before he had the time to be infected with that sickness and sadness in the heart of a gay boy. (p. 210)

The play has two minor gay characters, Bobby (aged seventeen) and an older man, Quentin, who has picked up the former on the road. Quentin has gone off the younger because he is not straight – he only desires straight boys:

> I only go for the straight trade. But this boy . . . look at him! Would you guess he was gay . . . I didn't, I thought he was straight. But I had an unpleasant surprise when he responded to my hand on his knee by putting his hand on mine. (p. 212)

Leona says of Quentin, talking to the boy: 'He wants to pay you, it's part of his sad routine' (p. 212). This particular situation – the gay man who cannot relate sexually to other gay men, and actually *wants* to pay for sex to ensure its impersonality – must stand as a powerful metaphor of self-contempt and an indicator of a total inability to develop mature relationships.

Quentin himself has a long speech about his gayness:

> There's a coarseness, a deadening coarseness, in the experience of most homosexuals. The experiences are quick, and hard, and brutal, and the pattern of them is practically unchanging. Their act of love is like the jabbing of a hypodermic needle to which they're addicted but which is more and more empty of real interest and surprise. This lack of variation and surprise in their . . . 'love life' . . . [*He smiles harshly*] spreads into other areas of . . . 'sensibility'? [*He smiles again.*] (p. 215)

Later in the speech he talks about smashing his car into a tree, not sure whether or not he meant to do it, and thus bringing into the play the classic suicide/homosexuality linkage which Williams has already used in *Streetcar*. The fact that Williams, apparently extrapolating from his own experience, impliedly insists that these are general truths about gay men, is a significant negative feature of his work.

* * *

In the second part of this chapter, I wish to consider some more general themes connected with sexuality. Williams's own search for love, resulting in his usually finding sensual gratification instead, appears in the plays as a preoccupation with the male figures as sexually attractive rather than loving or lovable. Indeed, we can go further and say that their sexual desirability is largely built on their not being lovable or solicitous. Stanley Kowalski, Brick, Val and Chance Wayne all treat the women with whom they are involved badly; they thereby become more desirable to the women within the plays. Estelle tells Serafina: 'A man that's wild is hard for a woman to hold, huh? But if he was tame – would the woman want to hold him? Huh?'[4]

Some heterosexual men and women in the audience will also be attracted by such male characters: the men because it reinforces notions of masculine dominance, the women because some of them will share Estelle's viewpoint. Some gay men will also read the male characters' behaviour as signalling a disengagement from women, and therefore heterosexuality itself. This latter point, although it might appear far-fetched, is underscored by such details as the male camraderie which exists between Stanley and his poker-playing friends and from which the 'womenfolk' are emphatically excluded.

Two literary/cultural traditions are involved here. The first is the idea that 'pure' male friendships are disrupted by women. From Polixenes and Leontes in *The Winter's Tale* (they want to be 'boy eternal') to the television detectives Starsky and Hutch hugging each other in brazenly homoerotic embraces (a daring 'taken back' and supposedly nullified by the men's girlfriends apearing in the background for two minutes every fifth episode for the purpose of guaranteeing the heterosexuality of the heroes), European culture is saturated in the notion that ideal male platonic friendships are destroyed by the intrusion of heterosexual desire.

The second tradition is that culture, refinement and kindness itself, in men, are seen as emasculating; that virility entails a kind of brutishness. In fiction, women are often forced to choose between these two types. In *Jane Eyre*, the powerful, rough-mannered Rochester ('manly') is counterpoised with the solicitous clergyman St John Rivers ('wimp'). Eliot's *Mill on the Floss* has a similar dichotomy, as does, perhaps most famously, Lawrence's *Daughters of the Vicar* (another clergyman, pale and ineffectual in his carpet slippers, 'like a little abortion', contrasted to the dour yokel miner, an icon of male beauty). Let us see how these two traditions appear in Williams.

The idea of a pure male friendship is at the heart of *Cat on a Hot Tin Roof*. Brick is no longer willing, or able, to make love to his wife because of the traumatic termination of his relationship with Skipper. (The name, of course, is suggestive of the masculine-dominated world of sport, which involves athleticism – that is, beauty – and 'healthy' male competitiveness.) Skipper kills himself when, after finally confiding on the phone to his friend that his love is not 'ideal' but sexual, Brick hangs up on him. (A closely similar betrayal occurs when Blanche DuBois rejects her husband when she discovers him in bed with another man, and the husband also kills himself.) In rejecting him thus, Brick has in effect killed his friend. His insistence that he is disgusted with the world, and has therefore taken to drink in order to forget, is a monstrous evasion. His father spells out the truth:

> This disgust with mendacity is disgust with yourself. You! – dug the grave of your friend and kicked him in it! – before you'd face the truth with him![5]

We can take this episode in several ways. The first is simply to make the observation, made by Brick himself, that human beings need lies and comfortable evasions. (Compare Amanda's insistence in *The Glass Menagerie* that nobody in the house must ever refer to Laura's lameness (= sexual undesirability).) The second is that these 'ideal' male friendships are seriously deficient if they crumble when one of the friends strays beyond conformist norms. The third is that Brick himself is refusing to come to terms with his own homosexuality. This last argument is simplistic; it represents a tendency amongst gay readers which, at its worst, seeks to find safety in numbers by seeing homosexuality as more widespread than is the case. It avoids the central issue: how, and under what circumstances, can men love men? That all men have a need to love other men I take for granted; that, as feminists have correctly and repeatedly pointed out, they are appallingly inept at doing so, I likewise believe. In Brick's case, what has made him take the extreme step of the treacherous betrayal of his friend, is that disgust with homosexuality which the play identifies as pathological. But that fear constantly invades relationships between two heterosexual men, creating a paranoia that expressions of love between men will somehow be 'tainted' by associations of homosexuality. That this point is also clearly part of the play's meaning is illustrated by Brick's and Skipper's behaviour before the revelation on the telephone. Brick tells his father that once in a while the two friends would put a hand on a shoulder and even, when sharing a hotel room, 'we'd reach across the space between the two beds and shake hands to say goodnight . . .'[6] Any man, the play surely tells us, who thinks that shaking hands with another man across the space between two single beds is a daring intimacy, is emotionally incomplete. To put this matter in cultural perspective, I should say that in Arabic countries (such as Tunisia, where I teach) men hug and kiss each other, and share a common bed, usually without the slighest desire or intention of any sexual intimacy. And lest it should be thought that this is the result of the oppressive seclusion of women in these societies, we should remember that such physical intimacies were a commonplace of pre-Second World War Britain – that is, before homosexuality was on the agenda, when it was unmentionable and sufficiently taboo a subject for it to be thought outrageous to infer homosexual desire on the basis of demonstrations of physical intimacies. This play, by design or not, shows that the victims of the taboo against same-sex expressions of love, verbal or physical, are heterosexual as well as homosexual. More specifically, and at the most obvious level, it also points out, in an age when very few people were 'out', the difficulty of identifying which men one could proposition. That is, we can easily imagine two gay men, in love with each other, shaking hands across the beds and afraid of going further out of fear that the other is heterosexual – a situation, *mutatis mutandis*, experienced by almost all the gay men I've met.

The second tradition – that of the desirability of the brutish male – is closely connected to the gay penchant for rough trade, whose essence is impersonal sex, and the fantasy of the male body as a fetishistic object rather than the housing of a person. (I should add that having created conditions in which full loving relationships between men are rendered practically impossible, leaving men in this period with outlets only in fugitive one-night stands and impersonal sex, heterosexuals then conclude that gay men are by nature promiscuous and unable to sustain stable relationships.) The tradition is best represented by Stanley Kowalski. Violent, drunken, unpredictable and insensitive, it is almost as if these characteristics are an appropriately pleasing complement to his hard musculature. He is contemptuous of Blanche's mock-modest flirtatious fishing for compliments: 'I never met a woman that didn't know if she was good-looking or not without being told, and some of them give themselves credit for more than they've got',[7] he tells her. One approach to Stanley's relationship with Blanche is that it shows Williams as misogynistic. Here is a self-deceiving, age-obsessed, semi-hysterical, mendacious, promiscuous, snobbish woman of faded gentility pretending immunity to Stanley's sexual charms. On another level, it could be seen as a healthy corrective to the male-created myth that women do not have sexual desires. Here, with a vengeance, is someone practically overcome with an excess of sensuality; she has lost her teaching post at Laurel as a result of the scandal which this sexual appetite generated. She is the victim of society's disapproval – its rejection and abhorrence of female promiscuity – in the same way that Brick and Skipper are victims.

There is a further connection in the two cases. Brick betrays Skipper because of the latter's homosexuality. Blanche embarks on her life of reckless promiscuity after betraying, in a very similar way, her gay husband. He, too, like Skipper, kills himself as a result of her having rejected him.

In *Orpheus Descending*, the relationship between Val and Lady shares some similarity with the issues discussed in connection with Stanley and Blanche. Lady begins by hiring Val in her store, and emphasizing, disingenuously, that she's 'not interested in your perfect functions, in fact you don't interest me no more than the air you stand in'.[8] In fact, it has already been made clear that she is excited by the casual, suggestive sensuality of his talk. Williams has mastered this sort of dialogue superbly:

LADY . . . [*She puts the jacket on as if to explore it*] It feels warm all right.
VAL. It's warm from my body, I guess . . .
LADY. You must be a warm-blooded boy . . .
VAL. That' right . . .

LADY. Well, what in God's name are you lookin' for around here?
VAL. Work.
LADY. Boys like you don't work.
VAL. What d'you mean by boys like me?
LADY. Ones that play the guitar and go around talkin' about how warm they are . . .
VAL. That happens t'be the truth. My temperature's always a couple degrees above normal the same as a dog's, it's normal for me the same as it is for a dog, that's the truth . . .[9]

The latent eroticism of this dialogue is enriched by its humour, which is largely lacking in *Streetcar*. Far from being a mere adjunct, it gives the exchange a poignancy. When she says, 'You must be a warm-blooded boy . . .' she is disguising her desire by means of a mild ironic mockery. In fact, she is raising the sexual heat of the exchange. Similarly, her 'Boys like you don't work' is spoken in the full knowledge that she will have to explain its meaning, which leads to her being allowed to repeat the 'warm' theme. So at the same time as raising the heat of the exchange, she is pretending to pour scorn on his representing himself to her as sexually charged. This is clearly akin to Blanche's sexual dishonesty. Both plays begin with the women trying to put down the men, only to be deeply humiliated later when the men confront the women with the latter's sexual desires. In Act Two of *Orpheus*, Val is urged by Lady to tell her what he means by saying he can see through her. She insists on knowing, yet is counting on his avoiding any painful home truths – a fact made clear by her violent reaction afterwards – but actually he does not spare her:

– A not so young and not so satisfied woman, that hired a man off the highway to do double duty without paying overtime for it . . . I mean a store clerk days and a stud nights . . .[10]

When Val then tries to walk out on her, all restraint and pretense vanishes:

[*She catches her breath; rushes to intercept him, spreading her arms like a crossbar over the door.*]

> LADY. NO, NO, DON'T GO . . . I NEED YOU!!! TO LIVE . . . TO GO ON LIVING!!!![11]

Lady and Blanche, then, are examples of sexual dishonesty; a point emphasised in the ironic connotations of their names, which suggest decorum and purity respectively.

This sexual dishonesty is also at the root of Serafina's character in *The Rose Tattoo.* Once again, we see the struggle within the heroine's personality between elegance and refinement – the emphasis on her 'aristocratic' marriage, and (? ironic) stage directions telling us, for example, that she has 'the dignity of a baronessa'[12] – and her preoccupation with the sensuality of her marriage. As in the other plays, 'love' in its wider sense, including rapport of personality and the associated traditional moral virtues (self-denial, solicitude, and so on), is hardly suggested. Relationships – and it is as if Williams challenges us to accept the unpalatable 'truth' of this, though indeed it is a very partial sort of truth – hinge on sensuality. All other advantages are trivial or spurious.

The play's strength and weakness arise from its having, effectively, this single focus. Whereas desire is a significant part of *Orpheus, Streetcar* and *Menagerie,* in this play it is emphasised almost to the exclusion of anything else.

William's version of sensuality here, as elsewhere, is both direct and metaphorical. Directly, Serafina explains insistently and at length why, after her husband's death, she has chosen celibacy:

> When I think of men I think about my husband. My husband was a Sicilian. We had love together every night of the week, we never skipped one, from the night we was married till the night he was killed in his fruit truck on that road there![13]

There is an emotional force here, a quality of memory and tenacity in relation to it, which we are invited to respect. But the words are partly undercut by irony. The second sentence we can hear with conviction, but also as typical of a particularly risible form of stereotyping, all the more interesting as it shows a woman 'intellectually collaborating' with a set of facile sexual assumptions: the identification of passion in the male rather/much more than in the female; the idea of the hot-blooded

Southerner; and the association of sexuality and crime (Sicilian = criminal; the husband's dangerous and illegal, therfore 'virile', smuggling). Also, 'We had love' rather than 'We made love' emphasises impersonality and eroticism. (We can compare Chance's comment to Princess about the former's girlfriend: 'I was just two years older, we had each other that early.'[14]) All these features taken together suggest to some readers that Williams has simply and implausibly attached a gay sensibility to a female character in order to express those feelings and ideas which, if expressed as overtly gay, would not be acceptable.

A second feature of Serafina's attitude is an élitist one. She despises Flora and Bessie – 'good time girls' flirting sillily with 'some middle-aged men, not young, not full of young passion, but getting a pot belly on him and losing his hair and smelling of sweat and liquor'[15] – because, in contrast to them, she had 'the best': 'Not the third best and not the second best, but the *first* best, the only *best*! – So now I stay here and am satisfied now to remember . . .'[16] (Once again the strength of utterance is undercut; in this case, by the comic disorder of the grammar.) The élitism also surfaces in her insistence on the land-owning status of her husband.

When Serafina first meets Alvaro, she only begins to take an interest in him – which, in Williams, means a sexual interest – when his profile outlined against the light brings back to her with a stab the memory of the body of her husband. One of the play's messages is that Serafina's self-entombment in the supposedly ideal past, is life-denying, and that to choose *second*-best – that is, Alvaro, with her husband's body but the mind and face of a clown – is a valid and wise choice. She of course does this, but only after the ideal past has been unmasked as a sham, through her discovery of her husband's adultery. Her smashing of the urn containing the husband's ashes represents her liberation from that past.

Before that liberation, Serafina is sexually and emotionally deprived, and takes it out on her daughter by means of an authoritarian attitude. Particularly, she fights an inevitably doomed battle against her daughter's developing sexual feelings, and her love for the sailor Jack. (Once again, the young, beautiful and virginal sailor is a homoerotic icon available to some members of the audience.) Only when she faces the reality of her own sexual position – that the ideal marriage was not ideal, and that she can begin to live again, certainly more honestly, with a man not available for unhealthy deification – can she consent to the sexual happiness of her daughter. What is recorded in this play are the inroads made by sexual jealousy, the extraordinary force of that emotion, and its ability to produce monstrous and extreme actions. In the case of *Orpheus* and *Sweet Bird of Youth*, these actions include murder. For many, the sexual pleasure of others is unbearable, rendering them literally murderous. An understanding of this seems to me especially acute among gay writers.

I spoke of both direct and metaphorical modes of communicating Williams's ideas on sensuality. One of the play's chief metaphors is, of course, that of the rose tattoo. The phrase is a kind of oxymoron; for 'tattoo' suggests social defiance, sailors, working-class eroticism, whereas 'rose', both in its sense here of the flower, but also, more strongly, in the parallel evocation of the colour pink, is altogether softer and 'feminine'. The rose itself is of course a symbol of love, and with its dual attributes of blossom and thorns, presents both the beautiful and painful aspects of love. Williams perhaps wants to unite, in his depictions of the husband, the brute/wimp dichotomy already discussed above; the passionate, criminal Sicilian is associated with a 'feminine' colour.

But pink is not only 'feminine' but gay. Long before it had become a political colour for the gay movement, it was associated, particularly where clothes were concerned, with homosexuality. Men are still alive today who would not, for example, wear a pink shirt for this reason. The rose (as colour) motif thus combines a suggestive softer side to the brutish male, and tantalising gay associations. This ambiguity also appears in the scene in which Estelle orders a rose-coloured shirt – not only that, but to be made of silk – from Serafina:

> SERAFINA [*involuntarily*]. Che bella stoffa! – Oh, that would be wonderful stuff for a lady's blouse or for a pair of pyjamas!
> ESTELLE. I want a man's shirt made with it.
> SERAFINA. Silk this colour for a *man*?
> ESTELLE. This man is wild like a gypsy.[17]

The gypsy analogy continues the idea of a man fundamentally

strong, but sensitive and soft also; and, like Jack the sailor, with a ring in his ear.

It is not clear how this gay/feminine equivocation works. The most fatuous response, which one sometimes hears, is that these heterosexual men are 'really' gay. It is understandable that in a world full of men denying the varieties of their sexual desires in an attempt to cram themselves uncomfortably into the fixed patterns society allows, readers should interpret the slightest signs of sexual ambiguity as indicators of bisexuality or homosexuality. A more interesting response is to see the play as saying that masculinity is not, and should not be seen to be, compromised by the 'feminine'.

The last play I wish to discuss is *Sweet Bird of Youth*. The hero, Chance Wayne, shares the status of transient which we saw in Val; both men suggest, to the audience and to themselves (especially Chance), a huge gap between potential and actual achievement. Both are forced to work at menial jobs whilst dreaming of something infinitely better; as is the case with Tom Wingfield, and, indeed, the early life of the author himself.

This sense of transience is heightened by moral disengagement. Chance, as his name suggests, does not make rational inferences about his repeated failures to succeed in Hollywood; he simply does not see that he lacks ability, and is determined to try repeatedly until successful, by whatever means. These include attempting to rig a beauty contest, and acting as a gigolo. In blaming 'chance' rather than assuming personal responsibility (in this, he is a kind of anti-existentialist) he is seen as attractively free of the stifling conventions of mainstream society. Heavenly certainly sees him as passive in this sense, for in explaining his failure to 'make himself big', she says: 'The right doors wouldn't open, and so he went in the wrong ones . . .'[18] This attitude of Chance's is partly attractive because it is 'mean', thus linking Chance to the 'brute' type represented by Stanley Kowalski.

The 'meanness' is marked. Chance deserts his dying mother without keeping in touch with her during her last days; he then concludes that 'She never had any luck'[19] as though the misfortune of dying alone were an accident of fate. He gives a flip self-exoneration when telling Princess: 'all my vices were caught from other people'[20] The central vacuity of his life – which is the pursuit of Hollywood glamour and wealth – is turned into a significant irony, for he himself represents, to

Heavenly, and even to the audience in some sense, something positive: youthful defiance, 'cool', a tempting amorality. This last quality is why he is so suitable as a companion for Princess; he has no debilitating qualms about selling his services, and being entirely and ruthlessly, like her, selfish. At different times in the play, each abandons the other without flinching, when they feel that it is not in their own interests. They are both, in Princess's word, 'monsters'.[21]

So here is the opposite of that innocent, boy–girl, mutually respecting intense love seen in Jack and Rosa. Princess is paying for raw sensuality. For her, sex is the 'only one way to forget these things I don't want to remember . . .'[22] But even here, there is a longing for some sexual illusion. She summons Chance to her arms at the end of Act One with: 'Now get a little sweet music on the radio and come here to me and make me almost believe that we're a pair of young lovers without any shame.'[23]

The point is that Chance ought to see that Princess, the pathetic, dream-wrecked drug-taking, lustful 'monster' is what he is becoming himself. (His drug habit is already established.) That is, he craves to enter the portals of that Hollywood where Princess is already ensconced – with hideous consequences. The gates to nowhere are those with the heaviest guards.

The sexual liaison between Chance and Princess, being mercenary, unloving and sordid, is far more real to us than the idealistic one with Heavenly. (The latter's name gives weight to this feeling.) Chance locates amorous sublimity in the past, which has all the luscious unreality of Hollywood. It can't have been (or can it?) that good, we ask ourselves. The photograph of fifteen-year-old Heavenly provokes Chance's memory: 'This was taken with the tide coming in. The water is just beginning to lap over her body like it desired her like I did and still do and will always, always.'[24] This kind of love, whether exaggerated or not, is for Williams indispensable to genuine human fulfilment. Those not thus fulfilled wreak, therefore, a terrible vengeance, as the fate of Val and Chance illustrates. (The first castrated, the other presumably severely beaten or even killed.) The sexual desirability of these men is, by implication, a reproach to those who lack it:

> Princess, the great difference between people in this world is not between the rich and the poor or the good and the evil, the

biggest of all differences in this world is between the ones that had or have pleasure in love and those that haven't and hadn't any pleasure in love, but just watched it with envy, sick envy. The spectators and the performers. I don't just mean ordinary pleasure or the kind you can buy, I mean great pleasure, and nothing that's happened to me or to Heavenly since can cancel out the many long nights without sleep when we gave each other such pleasure in love as very few people can look back on in their lives . . .[25]

In the lives of Lady, Serafina, Blanche, Val and Chance, there is a memory of, and a desperate struggle to get back to, a personal sexual idyll. The results of that attempt to return vary considerably. In Lady, the desire is chanelled into an unseemly and undignified seduction of Val, and the setting up of the confectionery, which can only, in fact, be a pale imitation of her father's orchard, which it is meant, in her mind, to replace. Serafina's ability to shed the chains of the past and accept another man – clearly Alvaro is not 'the best' – is, for all its psychological practicality, a compromise; Blanche's denial of her past in Laurel is disastrous; Val's disillusionment with 'love' leads quickly to his taking up prostitution, and Chance becomes a gigolo.

Two forces, in particular, work against them all. One is the clock. The close of *Sweet Bird of Youth* focuses on the ticking of the clock, and Chance comparing time to a rat gnawing away at its own foot, caught in a trap. Once it has gnawed itself free, it is disabled from escape; the whole process becomes futile in retrospect. The second force dooming these characters is desire itself. As Williams puts it, speaking personally:

All my life I have been haunted by the obsession that to desire a thing or to love a thing intensely is to place yourself in a vulnerable position, to be a possible, if not a probable, loser of what you most want.[26]

8

Yukio Mishima: *Confessions of a Mask*

Yukio Mishima (1925–70) was born in Tokyo, the son of a senior government official. He was a delicate and precocious child, and from adolescence was deeply affected by pictures of physical violence and pain, and especially by Guido Reni's Saint Sebastian *– all of which is reflected in* Confessions of a Mask*. During the Second World War he met the writer Yasunari Kawabata; this was the beginning of a lifelong friendship. He entered Tokyo University to study law in 1944, and in February 1945 was conscripted for war service. He did not see active service although the war experience affected him profoundly, and laid the foundation of the death worship which he later developed. He graduated in law in 1947, spent one year as a civil servant, and then turned to full-time writing. After a depressing visit to New York in 1957, he developed a philosophy which he called 'active nihilism', an element of which was the idealising of suicide as the ultimate existentialist gesture – a gesture which he was to perform in 1970, at the headquarters of the Japanese defence forces. He was married and had two children, but it is clear that he was homosexual and not bisexual.*

Mishima is in the tradition of Byron, Wilde, Genet and Orton; the acts and preoccupations of his writings are more than usually reflective of his own life. *Confessions of a Mask*[1] is widely thought to be especially closely autobiographical. My approach in this chapter will be to discuss the *Confessions* in relation to certain aspects of his life and his political ideology.

Mishima was born in 1925, and was therefore a youth when war broke out. During his adolescence, he was convinced that the war would claim his life; he enjoyed, and he stressed this time and again in his writings, the anticipation of death. The spirit of militarism invested his being in the highest degree. It might therefore seem an oddity that he was guilty of faking illness at the examination for entry into the army. However, the explanation that emerged much later in his life, expressed in his essay *Sun and Steel*,[2] was that a glorious death was impossible without a beautiful body. But he did not have one; his body was rather puny and sickly. Therefore death had to be postponed. Later in life, his narcissistic obsession led him to devote many hours to body building. (His delight in posing nearly naked for erotic photographs reminds us of Joe Orton, though the latter's interest was nowhere near so intense as Mishima. Also, Mishima was keen to have the photographs published.) It was with an impressively muscled body that Mishima committed *seppuku* in 1970.

His real name was Kimitaké Hiraoka, and as a child he was exceedingly bright at his studies. When he left school the Emperor himself presented him with an award for distinguishing himself. Extremely precocious, his first long work, *The Forest in Full Bloom*, came out in 1941 when Mishima was only sixteen. As a schoolboy he achieved top grades in all academic subjects (except physics) but was poor in physical exercises and martial arts – something he of course rectified much later in life when he took up kendo very seriously, as well as body building. According to his friend Henry Stokes, 'For the rest of his life he attempted to compensate for his [physical] frailty by prodigious actions.'[3]

An especially important detail about his early life was that he was cooped up as a child with his grandmother, who more or less stole Mishima from his mother and forced him to stay with her for hours and hours as she lay in her sick bed. Mishima was rarely allowed outside the house. This exclusion from the outside world, which affected the child strongly, no doubt gave rise to the following very poignant composition, written when he was seven, illustrating the general prohibition about going on outings, and anticipating the theme of lonely enforced individuality which figures so conspicuously in his later work:

'Enoshima Excursion'

I did not go on the school outing.
When I woke up that day I thought: 'Now everyone must be at Shinjuku Station, on the train.'
I easily think of things like that.

> I went to my grandmother and my mother. I wanted so much to go. Just at that moment they would all have arrived at Enoshima.
> I wanted to go so much because I had never been there.
> I was thinking of it from morning to evening
> When I went to bed I had a dream.
> I *did* go to Enoshima with everyone else, and I played there very happily. But I could not walk at all. There were rocks..
> Then I woke up.[4]

Most of his adult life was spent in writing, although he also appeared in gangster films and erotic photographs in order to satisfy his narcissism. After the war, he was generally regarded as being sympathetic to the left, though he was not directly involved in politics. However, from the early 1960s until his death by ritual suicide in 1970 he became increasingly right wing. These views were expressed publicly at meetings as well as through his creative writing. At the heart of Mishima's ideology was the role of the Emperor, and this role was very similar to today's Arab nations' view of the ideal head of state: that is a strong leader aware of the glories of the past and determined to act resolutely, even ruthlessly, in order to fulfil what is perceived as the historical destiny of the people. The ideology is strongly authoritarian, patriotic, traditionalist, nationalist and xenophobic, and relies very heavily on the cult of the leader. It embraces all aspects of life, even the most personal. For example, Mishima believed that love could not exist between two people in modern societies without a god or an emperor; but with a god or emperor, their love can flourish as their love is based on a shared esteem for the superior being.

Inevitably, such a society thrives on violence and the idea of violence. Mishima told Stokes that he felt kinship with his student enemies on the left because he and they shared 'a rigorous ideology and a taste for physical violence'.[5] Authoritarianism, violence, and eroticism all came together. For example, one of Mishima's favourite works, the *Hagakure*, an eighteenth-century account of *samurai* ethics, explains the relationship between *samurai* warriors in terms of love.

Mishima himself set up a paramilitary force of young men, the *Takenokai*, who were dressed in suggestive and very becoming uniforms which he had designed himself. (Because of his celebrity and his contacts within the defence force, the *Jieitai,* he was given official permission for all this.) The formation of the *Takenokai* centred on university students. The nature of the organisation can be gauged by the bizarre blood ceremony which took place in 1967 at the offices of a rightist magazine, and described to Mishima's father by someone who was there. About twelve people were present:

> On a piece of paper [Mishima] wrote in Chinese ink: 'We hereby swear to be the foundation of Kokoku Nippon [Imperial Japan].' Then he cut his little finger with a pen-knife and asked eveyone else to follow his example. They dripped blood from their fingers into a cup, all standing round, until it was brimful; then each signed his name on the piece of paper, dipping a brush into the cup and signing in blood. . . . Some of the people felt faint and one had to rush out of the door to vomit. Mishima then suggested that they should drink the blood . . . he picked up the glass and asked: 'Is anyone here ill? None of you have VD?' All seemed well. He called for a salt cellar and flavoured the cup; then he drank from it. The others followed his example. 'What a fine lot of Draculas,' said Mishima, looking round at the youths with their red mouths and teeth, laughing his raucous laugh.[6]

The nature of such an organisation, combined with the cult of emperor worship, inevitably led to Mishima having a contempt for those people who, however sympathetic some of them might be, could not give themselves wholeheartedly to such a zealous creed. At the end of his life, he wrote in the preface to a biography of the writer Zenmei Hasuda about his hatred of Japanese intellectuals, a hatred shared with Hasuda:

> [Hasuda's] fury was directed at Japanese intellectuals, the strongest enemy within the nation. It is astonishing how little the character of modern intellectuals in Japan has changed, i.e. their cowardice, sneering, 'objectivity', rootlessness, dishonesty, flunkeyism, mock gestures of resistance, self-importance, inactivity, talkativeness, and readiness to eat their words.[7]

In choosing material for his novels, Mishima was inspired by certain famous historical incidents which for him involved the assertion of traditional Japanese virtues. One of these was the Shinpuren Incident (1877), inspired by hostile reaction to a government decree ordering *samurai* no longer to wear their swords and for them to cut off their topknots. The rebels believed in *Sonno Joi* (the two chief ideas here were to revere the Emperor and expel the barbarian), hated foreigners and were very pious. Such was their hostility to modernity that when forced to walk under electric power lines, they covered their heads with white fans. The rebellion itself was, for Mishima, a noble failure – most of the rebels who were not killed in the fighting committed *seppuku*.

Another more recent but similar event, the NI NI Roku Incident, occurred in 1936; Mishima's story 'Yokoku' ('Patriotism') is based on it. A group of rebels killed three members of the government, claiming to be in support of the Emperor but opposed to his wicked advisers. Hirohito ordered them to surrender, which they did. Mishima supported the rebel officers and wrote twice more about the incident: in the play *Toka no Kiku*, and the elegy for the war dead, 'Eirei no Koe' ('The Voices of the Heroic Dead', 1966).

In 'Patriotism', the rebel lieutenant commits *seppuku* and his wife, following him, stabs herself in the throat, having arranged the folds of her dress in such a way that she will not be found in an indecorous position. Mishima writes:

> To choose the place where one dies is also the greatest joy in life. And such a night as the couple had was their happiest. . . . the love of these two reaches to an extremity of purity. . . . Somewhere I obtained the conviction that if one misses one's night one will never have another opportunity to achieve a peak of happiness in life. Instrumental in this conviction were my experiences during the war, my reading of Nietzsche during the war. . . . Their [the rebels'] purity, bravery, youth and death qualified them as mythical heroes; and their failures and deaths made them true heroes in this world.[8]

We can see from this that death, and especially death in battle or ritual suicide, excited the imagination and fervour of Mishima, who throughout his writings imbued it with both eroticism and nobility. It was natural that he should have looked back with particular affection to the group *Nippon Roman-ha* ('Japanese Romanticists' is a loose translation), which was active in the 1930s and whose members believed in holy war, the Emperor, the superior destiny of Japan and the superiority of its people, the warrior ethic, and the value of destruction and self-destruction, which latter would be followed by reincarnation. (Stokes thinks that Mishima himself did not actually believe in reincarnation.) *Death was the ultimate value.* Members included Zenmei Hasuda (see above), Yojuro Yasuda (a critic), and Shizuo Ito (a poet, with whom the young Mishima had corresponded). It was influenced by German Romanticism and centred on a magazine edited by Yasuda called *Nippon Roman.*

Death is the ultimate value partly because, following the classical Roman tradition, it can be summoned at any time. No man is a slave because he does not have to stay in the world. We are free because not even the most powerful tyrant can prevent our voluntary departure, through suicide. It is the opposite of the curious Western hypothesis that suicide is pathological. By the summer of 1970, just before his own suicide, Mishima was describing *seppuku* as 'the ultimate masturbation'.[9]

In 'Patriotism', Mishima describes *seppuku* in enormous and gruesome detail – probably the most detailed description in Japanese literature. (Mishima was the only Japanese novelist of repute to have written about *seppuku.*) Blood, grease, vomiting, the slithery entrails with their raw stench were all included; ending with 'It would be difficult to imagine a more heroic sight than that of the lieutenant at this moment, as he mustered his strength and flung back his head.'[10] In his final work, the tetralogy called *The Sea of Fertility,* Mishima returns to the theme of ritual suicide in the death of characters such as Isao.

It has always to be remembered, in contrast to Western practice, that Japanese suicide was commonly chosen for reasons of honour. Hasuda, who was an important Japanese writer who felt quite close personally to Mishima, murdered his commanding officer during the war for criticising the Emperor and then shot himself in the head; he was a member of *Nippon Roman-ha.* Yasunari Kawabata, the first Japanese to get the Nobel Prize (in 1968), something Mishima himself coveted and had several times been tipped for, gassed himself in 1972. Indeed, since the beginning of the century, suicide by writers was common: Bizan Kawakami (1908); Takeo Arishima (1923?); Akutagawa (1927);

Shinichi Makino (1936); Osamu Dazai (1948); Tamiki Hara (1951); Michio Kato (1953); Sakae Kubo (1958); Ashihei Hino (1960).

If death could be erotic and noble, it was only thus by dint of effort. The body had to be prepared, made strong and beautiful – hence the narcissism. The erotic photographs taken by the fashionable Eiko Hosoe show Mishima stripped naked in a garden with a white rose in his mouth; or, again nude, on a rocky foreshore. These appeared in the album *Barakei.* Mishima also appears, in a photograph taken by Kishin Shinoyama, as Saint Sebastian, after the painting by Guido Reni. (It is the Reni picture which, in *Confessions,* inspires the narrator's first ejaculation.) Other photos of Mishima by Shinoyama include one of the writer in boots, black jock strap and sailor cap, leaning against a huge motorcycle. Mishima also acted in a gangster film, *Karakkaze Yaro* (*A Dry Fellow*). At the start of the film we see him stripped to the waist in a prison yard; it is a hooligan part. The film ends with his murder.

Mishima was not prepared to accept the decay of the body, the temple of immortal longings. A passage in *Sun and Steel* referring to the muscles of the body runs:

> Their one flaw was that they were too closely involved with the life processes, which decreed that they should decline and perish with the decline of life itself.[11]

Speaking *in propria persona,* Mishima said on the same subject:

> . . . the body is doomed to decay, just like the complicated motor of a car. I for one do not, will not, accept such a doom. This means that I do not accept the course of Nature.[12]

One way out of this dilemma, albeit a temporary one, was to engage in body building and kendo and other pursuits which kept that body relatively young. In this regard, it is characteristic of Mishima that, in 1956, he should join a team of local youths to carry the *omikoshi* (Shinto shrine) for the summer festival. (We come across this in *Confessions.*) He wears a *hachimaki* (headband) as he and the students were to do on the day of his suicide.

The other option is to destroy the body at the peak of its beauty. He wrote about this before he did it himself. For example, in *Sun and Steel*:

> The romantic impulse that had formed an undercurrent in me from boyhood on, and that made sense only as the *destruction* of classical perfection, lay waiting within me. . . . Specifically, I cherished a romantic impulse towards death, yet at the same time I required a strictly classical body as its vehicle; a peculiar sense of destiny made me believe that the reason why my romantic impulse towards death remained unfulfilled in reality was the immensely simple fact that I lacked the necessary physical qualifications. A powerful, tragic frame and sculpturesque muscles were indispensable in a romantically noble death. Any confrontation between weak, flabby flesh and death seemed to me absurdly inappropriate. Longing at eighteen for an early demise, I felt myself unfitted for it. I lacked, in short, the muscles suitable for a dramatic death. And it deeply offended my romantic pride that it should be this unsuitability that had permitted me to survive the war.'[13]

Hence his faking illness at the famous army medical in 1945.

Death was not simply for Mishima a terminal event, something to look forward to as one approached it and which, after its occurrence, placed the recently ended life in a special perspective. All that was true, but death also meant quasi-sexual pleasure. His novels – for example *The Middle Ages* (1946) and *Spring Snow* (1969) – are full of violent deaths. His modern Nō and Kabuki theatre pieces are also violent: for example, his last theatrical work, *Chinsetsu Yumiharizuki* (1969), has a woman torturing a naked male captive by drilling holes in his body with an awl. For Mishima, pain was always exciting:

> As my body acquired muscle, and in turn strength, there was gradually born within me a tendency towards the positive acceptance of pain, and my interest in physical suffering deepened. Even so, I would not have it believed that this development was a result of the workings of my imagination. My discovery was made directly, with my body.[14]

To the Westerner, there is always a degree of astonishment that a writer of great sensitivity and culture, a thoroughgoing intellectual, could allow himself to be seduced by what might well appear a manic obsession. This would be to fail to realise that the ideal *samurai* pursued his life and death according to the tradition of *Bunburyodo,* the dual way of literature (*Bun*) and the sword (*Bu*) (*ryodo* = dual way). In English literature, one has to go back to the Renaissance, and figures like Sir Philip Sydney, to see this blend of artistic sensitivity and martial enthusiasm.

The two emblems expressing Japanese attitudes most directly are the chrysanthemum and the sword. (At the time of writing, August 1990, I have just received a letter from Tokyo with two postage stamps; one shows a traditional suit of armour, the other a chrysanthemum.) During Mishima's lifetime, Westerners in his view concentrated on the flower and forgot the sword. He frequently referred with approval to Ruth Benedict's book, *The Chrysanthemum and the Sword*[15] because he felt she had understood the dual nature of Japanese society better than most Westerners. In a speech on 3 November 1969, he referred to the book and said:

> After the war the balance between these two was lost. The sword has been ignored since 1945. My ideal is to restore the balance. To revive the tradition of the samurai, through my literature and my action.[16]

Two months earlier, in an interview in *The* [*London*] *Times,* Mishima said that culture 'must embrace lightness and darkness equally'.[17]

In occasional moments during his life, and perhaps most supremely at the time of his death, Mishima believed that he had achieved *Bunburyodo.* Take, for example, this description of combat exercises with his *Takenokai* on Mount Fuji. It is evening and the weary youths assemble:

> After a long talk about how to command the attack squad, one of our members, a young man from Kyoto, brought out a flute in a beautiful damask bag. It was the type of flute used for Court music ever since the ninth century, and only very few people can play it nowadays. This lad had been studying it for about a year. . . . Now he began playing for us. It was a beautiful and moving melody that reminded me of the heavily bedewed autumn fields and of the Shining Prince Genji who had danced to this very music. As I listened in sheer rapture, it crossed my mind that for the first time in the post-war years the two Japanese traditions had come happily together, if only for a

> fleeting moment – the tradition of elegance and that of the *samurai*. It was this union that I had sought in the depth of my heart.[18]

In *Sun and Steel*, one of his most important essays and written two years before his death, he speaks of the 'ultra-erotic' nature of suicide. He goes on:

> No moment is so dazzling as when everyday imaginings concerning death and danger and world destruction are transformed into duty. . . . To keep death in mind from day to day, to focus each moment upon inevitable death, to make sure one's worst forebodings coincided with one's dreams of glory.

In an epilogue to the essay he describes a test flight in an F104 jet fighter:

> Erect-angled, the F104, a sharp silver phallus, pointed into the sky. Solitary, spermatozoon-like. I was installed within. Soon, I should know how the spermatozoon felt at the instant of ejaculation.[19]

Mishima completed his tetralogy, *The Sea of Fertility*, in 1970. On the same day as he placed the completed typescript on the hall table of his home, ready to be submitted to the publishers, he went to the headquarters of the Japanese defence forces with members of his own private force for a prearranged meeting. The group held the commanding officer captive on arrival, and demanded that all the soldiers on the base be assembled below the window of the CO's office so that Mishima could address the troops from the balcony. Some unsuccessful attempts were made to storm the room where the CO was held, but the attackers were beaten back, and sustained injuries. Mishima spoke to the troops about the necessity of resisting the treacherous modern ways of the army and returning to an emperor-based, militaristic tradition. He was ridiculed and laughed at at such volume that on an existing amateur recording of the speech, one can hardly hear his words for the din. He went back into the CO's office and committed *seppuku*.

Perhaps Mishima seriously believed that a nation-wide insurrection, beginning with soldiers whom he had worked up to a rebellion like that of NI NI Roku in 1936, would ensue as a result of his actions. But this is extremely unlikely. His real motive seems to have been to provide a suitably dramatic setting for his 'noble' death, a death he had desired for so long. The evidence for this is that, from Mishima's point of view, the moment was ideal. He was surrounded by his most favoured, hero-worshipping acolytes. One of them, Morita, may even have been his lover; but if not, he was certainly very close to Mishima and a sharer in his aspirations. The group had anticipated the need for suicide by bringing with them all the ritual paraphernalia of *seppuku* – the cloths, the swords, the *hachimaki*. Like the woman in 'Patriotism' who arranged her clothes decorously before stabbing herself in the throat, Mishima had provided himself and fellow-suicide Morita with cotton wool for their anuses so that they would not soil themselves during their deaths. In the event, Mishima knelt down and gashed open his stomach with the ritual short sword; then, following tradition, Morito cut off his head. Morito in turn knelt down and cut himself open, but he was not so lucky with his own decapitator, who repeatedly hacked at him without giving a clean and definitive stroke to the neck. He was finished off by a more stalward swordsman. And so perished one of Japan's most celebrated writers.

In the catalogue of an exhibition about his life and work (at the Tobu department store) Mishima divided his life into various rivers; in the section called 'The River of Action' he wrote about himself thus:

> The river of action gives me the tears, the blood, the sweat that I never begin to find in the River of Writing. In this new river I have encounters of soul with soul without having to bother about words. This is also the most destructive of all rivers, and I can well understand why few people approach it. . . . it brings no wealth nor peace, it gives no rest. Only let me say this: I, born a man and alive as a man, cannot overcome the tempation to follow the course of this River.[20]

I should now like to look in some detail at *Confessions* to see how some of Mishima's preoccupations find a voice in his most personal work. This novel is regarded as closely autobiographical, and we know from later evidence and interviews that many of the events described in it occurred in more or less the same way in Mishima's own life.

At the beginning of the novel, the first-person narrator, looking back to his childhood at the age of four, describes the first stirrings of a defiled eroticism. It is his encounter with the night-soil man (that is, the man who collects human excrement in buckets):

> . . . for me he represented my first revelation of a certain power, my first summons by a certain strange and secret voice. It is significant that this was first manifested to me in the form of a night-soil man: excrement is a symbol for the earth, and it was doubtless the malevolent love of the Earth Mother that was calling to me.
>
> I had a presentiment then that there is in this world a kind of desire like stinging pain. Looking up at that dirty youth, I was choked by desire, thinking, 'I want to change into him,' thinking, 'I want to *be* him.' I can remember clearly that my desire had two focal points. The first was his dark-blue 'thigh-pullers', the other his occupation. The close-fitting jeans plainly outlined the lower half of his body, which moved lithely and seemed to be walking directly toward me. An inexpressible adoration for those trousers was born in me. I did not understand why. . . . I became possessed with the ambition to become a night-soil man. The origin of this ambition might have been partly in the dark-blue jeans, but certainly not exclusively so. . . .
>
> What I mean is that toward his occupation I felt something like a yearning for a piercing sorrow, a body-wrenching sorrow. His occupation gave me the feeling of 'tragedy' in the most sensuous meaning of the word. A certain feeling as it were of 'self-renunciation', a certain feeling of indifference, a certain feeling of intimacy with danger, a feeling like a remarkable mixture of nothingness and vital power. (pp. 12–13)

The idea of 'tragedy' which the narrator has in this episode is to recur over and over again. In a later occurrence, he sees a troop of soldiers passing by his house:

> The soldiers' odor of sweat – that odor like a sea breeze, like the air, burned to gold, above the seashore – struck my nostrils and

> intoxicated me. . . . it did gradually and tenaciously arouse within me a sensuous craving for such things as the destiny of soldiers, the tragic nature of their calling, the distant countries, they would see, *the ways they would die* . . . (p. 17, my italics)

It is of course death which terminates all tragedy, and the narrator's obsession with death is unrelenting. Vital to an understanding of the link between death and eroticism in this case is his long meditation on the death of Saint Sebastian, inspired by his having seen a reproduction of the famous painting of the saint's martyrdom (tied to a crucifix and shot to death with arrows) by Guido Reni. I have mentioned above that Mishima posed as Sebastian for a photograph, modelled on the Reni painting. It should be remembered that this painting, and others depicting the same event, have always attracted, and continue to attract, a great deal of interest amongst gay men. In these paintings, considering the well-developed musculature of the body, and the passive vulnerability of the saint in the face of the infliction of cruel injustice, gay men clearly see a personal resonance. The Saint Sebastian paintings take only a little further the provocatively erotic crucified Christ icons of Catholicism. It has always been a wonderful irony that in purveying their anti-carnal and anti-love message, the priests have created, in the crucifixes and paintings of such figures as Christ and Sebastian, an iconography of almost unparalleled homoerotic power. The narrator's Sebastian is both beautiful and doomed, two attributes constantly linked in Mishima's writing:

> His was not a fate to be pitied. . . . Rather was it proud and tragic, a fate that might even be called shining.
>
> When one considers well, it seems likely that many a time, even in the midst of a sweet kiss, a foretaste of the agony of death must have furrowed his brow with a fleeting shadow of pain. (p. 41)

Mishima was aware of the historical homoerotic resonance of the Sebastian paintings. In *Confessions,* the narrator refers to the sexologist Magnus Hirschfield's discussion of them, and goes on to add tellingly, on his own account, that 'in the overwhelming majority of cases of inversion [i.e. homosexuality], especially of congenital inversion, the inverted and sadistic impulses are inextricably entangled with each other' (p. 38). Thus does the narrator/Mishima extrapolate his own personal desires and apply them wholescale to the 'overwhelming majority'. It is one of the great interests of this novel that one sometimes comes across passages like this, which have an ironic flavour in that, at the very moment of describing and indeed celebrating some of the most taboo-ridden desires and fantasies, we are nevertheless offered a commentary on them which appears to be based on all the negative pathology-oriented heterosexist assumptions of established opinion.

This is of course not surprising, given the period in which Mishima was writing. But perhaps even more relevant is the fact that Mishima himself, in his writing, expresses a profound contradiction: that of the ultra-traditional, Emperor-loving conformist who nevertheless needs to articulate not only gay desire, almost by definition 'revolutionary' and destabilising of family-oriented societies in which heterosexuality is compulsory, but a sado-masochistic version of it. We can, in fact, identify something like the Faustian spirit of defiance in many of the narrator's thoughts and reactions, especially his attitude towards Omi. Omi is the school nonconformist, always wearing forbidden clothes or indulging in unspecified wrongdoing. He is a figure of mystery who has created around himself an aura of evil which is for the narrator extraordinarily enticing. Omi 'possessed an uncanny skill for clothing his wickedness in the fair name of revolt' (p. 46). For Mishima, as for Genet and Orton, to have gay desire is, effectively, to be an outlaw and therefore to be drawn towards the defiantly anti-conventional.

At the same time, both the narrator of *Confessions* and Mishima himself engaged in elaborate deception by entering into amorous relationships with women as part of a desire to fit into a strongly conformist society. Mishima actually got married. *Confessions* is strewn with metaphors of deception (not least in the book's title), and descriptions of the way the narrator manages to fool everybody into believing something which is not the case. He persists with his courtship of Sonoko despite his distaste for female kisses. Chieko's embrace is like something from Samuel Beckett:

Suddenly I felt something touch my forehead, and with it came

> a faint breath against my skin. I turned my head and gave a meaningless sigh. At that instant my unusually fevered breath became mingled with hers. My lips were covered by something heavy and greasy. Our teeth crashed together noisily. I was afraid to open my eyes and look. Then she grasped my cheeks firmly between her two cold hands. (p. 152)

Thus the contradictory impulses of rebellion, based, at least originally, on his forbidden sexual desire, and conformity, especially strong in Japanese culture, did battle in both the life and writings of Mishima.

The narrator's childhood reading includes as many fairy tales as he can get his hands on. He always dislikes the princesses and can be enthused only by the princes. The best princes were those who were doomed:

> I was all the fonder of princes murdered or princes fated for death. . . . I did not understand why, out of Wilde's numerous fairy tales, it was only the corpse of the young fisherman in 'The Fisherman and His Soul', washed up on the shore clasping a mermaid to his breast, that captivated me. (p. 22)

It is no great leap from a love of death in others to a love of one's own demise. Later on, as a youth, he 'shuddered with a strange delight at the thought of my own death' (p. 98) and, before that, he speaks of two contending forces within him, struggling for supremacy. The first is 'self-preservation', and the second 'was a compulsion toward suicide, that subtle and secret impulse to which a person often unconsciously surrenders himself' (pp. 58–9).

The fantastic nature of this death obsession is revealed during the war when the narrator discusses what happens to him when he allows himself to imagine that his whole family has been annihilated in an air raid, including himself: 'Just the thought that I might see the cruel deaths of my family, and that they might see mine, made a retching nausea rise in my chest' (p. 113). The emphasis is not on the pain or the grief, but on the notion of what is seemly. It is undignified to die messily, watched by others, with no hint of the noble. (We remember the woman suicide in 'Patriotism'.) The narrator knows exactly what sort of death will best suit his own longings:

> What I wanted was to die among strangers, untroubled, beneath a cloudless sky. And yet my desire differed from the sentiments of that ancient Greek who wanted to die under the brilliant sun. What I wanted was some natural, spontaneous suicide. I wanted a death like that of a fox, not yet well versed in cunning, that walks carelessly along a montain path and is shot by a hunter because of its own stupidity. (pp. 113–4)

If we consider the precise nature and circumstances of Mishima's own death, this passage is prophetic, especially in the idea of a combination of courage and stupidity.

What is most extraordinary about this novel is the frank honesty, and very often in the prose the lyrical beauty, with which sexual desire is analysed and discussed. Not all of it is based on pain. Much of it is quite routine, such as his masturbation fantasy of the school instructor as a Hercules, and the episode of auto-eroticism, in which he uses his own armpits as a masturbatory stimulus. He also registers the desire for 'rough trade', unspoiled by a civilising intellect: 'young toughs, sailors, soldiers, fishermen' are the desired objects (p. 56). Unfortunately, to relate to these erotic 'savages' requires in himself a suspension of reason which he is quite unable to bring about. Thus, he is permanently condemned to 'watching them from afar with impassioned indifference' (p. 56).

The more celebrated and graphically described sado-masochism is a taste which starts in adolescence, when the narrator notices that he has erections when seeing

> death and pools of blood and muscular flesh. Gory dueling scenes on the frontispieces of adventure-story magazines . . . young samurai cutting open their bellies, or of soldiers struck by bullets, clenching their teeth and dripping blood from between hands that clutched at khaki-clad breasts. (p. 34)

Mishima is a kind of oriental version of Genet; his vision of human life is, if anything, even darker. Both men celebrate the erotic in their writings, in a manner both direct and often painfully honest, and place it very firmly at the centre of their interest; but always representing it as guilty and soiled. Mishima is of course immensely popular with homophobic critics like Jeffrey Meyers because homosexuality is linked to guilt, darkness, obsession and pain. Like Genet, Mishima would have thought with contempt of the present civil rights' movement for lesbians and gays. For him, despite the elements of pain and violence, and lest anyone new to Mishima should have gained the impression that there is anything of raunchiness in the writing, the erotic is supremely aesthetic. The meditation on the martyred Sebastian has the languor and happy placidity of Dorian Gray examining old brocades or rare watercolours:

> It is not pain that hovers about his straining chest, his tense abdomen, his slightly contorted hips, but some flicker of melancholy pleasure like music. Were it not for the arrows with their shafts deeply sunk into his left armpit and right side, he would seem more a Roman athlete resting from fatigue, leaning against a dusky tree in a garden.
>
> The arrows have eaten into the tense, fragrant, youthful flesh and are about to consume his body from within with flames of supreme agony and ecstasy. But there is no flowing blood, nor yet the host of arrows seen in other pictures of Sebastian's martyrdom. Instead, two lone arrows cast their tranquil and graceful shadows upon the smoothness of his skin, like the shadows of a bough falling upon a marble stairway. (p. 37)

9

James Baldwin: *Another Country* and *Giovanni's Room*

James Baldwin (1924–87), an illegitimate child, was brought up in Harlem in New York, where his father was a Christian minister. He was the first of nine children. As a young teenager, Baldwin also became a preacher, and the oratorical style he then used influenced the prose he went on to write, in both essays and fiction. He travelled extensively in Europe, and settled for many years in France, and an implied or express comparison between Europe and the United States can frequently be found in his writing. Throughout his life he was a vigorous and outspoken campaigner against racism, but was generally secretive and closeted about his sexual life in public, and took no part in gay rights campaigns. As with Forster, this dramatically reduced the liberating force of the works.

Two of Baldwin's novels, *Another Country* and *Giovanni's Room*,[1] deal centrally with gay relationships and issues of sexuality. The first-named of these is one of the great novels of our century, and I hope to give some indication of this in the discussion below. The earlier work is interesting in its own right, but especially worth examining because it shows the author in the toils of certain prejudices from which, by the time of the later book, he had largely emancipated himself. Studying the two novels together is thus particularly interesting as it provides, amongst other things, a kind of chart of the author's intellectual, moral and aesthetic development.

Another Country starts with an account of hell. Rufus, destitute, filthy, tired and hungry, staggers out of a cinema near Times Square, the classic sleazy New York location: 'Entirely alone, and dying of it, he was part of an unprecedented multitude' (p. 6). Repeatedly, throughout the work, Baldwin offers these parallels between the individual histories of his characters and the general malaise of the whole of United States society.

The stress on the isolation of one man or woman reminds us of Genet; but not so the idea of applying it generally, so that all Americans are represented as in some sense radically alienated. As the novel unfolds, and we come to see that at the heart of it is a minute, painfully honest and perceptive commentary on the state of various human emotions, especially over matters of love, we realise that what distinguishes most of the novel's characters from the multitude which is evoked, usually with contempt, is the degree of awareness. The masses appear to eat, sleep and die without any of the existentialist anguish which is described in the experience of the fictional characters.

This central theme – that the novel's individuals are apart from the majority of society by virtue of their greater existentialist perception of their miserable plight, and that the multitude is in a state of ignorant mindlessness – is repeatedly emphasised. Scenes focusing on individual misery constantly refer also to the general herd. Thus, a street scene gives us a procession of faces all of which, even those of the children, 'held a sweet or poisonous disenchantment' (p. 93). We are told that most people do not really 'live' at all; they experience bad events as though '[they] had simply been stunned by the hammer' (p. 103). The ordinary, faithful, heterosexual couple are similarly described: 'There seemed to be very little between his father and his mother, very little, that is, beyond habit and courtesy and coercion . . .' (p. 158). Thinking of the bigots of Alabama, Eric considers 'the hideous obsequiousness of people who despised him but who did not dare to say so. They had long ago given up saying anything which they really felt, had given it up so long ago that they were now incapable of feeling anything which was not felt by a mob' (p. 160). And at Rufus's funeral, the preacher warns against condemning Rufus for taking his own life:

> I know a lot of people done took their own lives and they're walking up and down the streets today and some of them is preaching the gospel and some is sitting in the seats of the mighty. Now, you remember that. If the world wasn't so full of

> dead folks maybe those of us that's trying to live wouldn't have to suffer so bad. (p. 98)

Old friends lose their charm, are ground down in the mill of the conventional. Baldwin cannot reconcile himself to this, finds it awful:

> There was something frightening about the aspect of old friends, old lovers, who had, mysteriously, come to nothing. It argued the presence of some cancer which had been operating in them, invisibly, all along and which might, now, be operating in oneself. Many people had vanished, of course, had returned to the havens from which they had fled. But many others were still visible, had turned into lushes or junkies or had embarked on a nerve-rattling pursuit of the perfect psychiatrist; were vindictively married and progenitive and fat; were dreaming the same dreams they had dreamed ten years before, clothed these in the same arguments, quoted the same masters; and dispensed, as they hideously imagined, the same charm they had possessed before their teeth began to fail and their hair began to fall. They were more hostile now than they had been, this was the loud, inescapable change in their tone and the only vitality left in their eyes. (pp. 25–6)

Vivaldo is a character who, unlike Richard, refuses to change with age; or perhaps one should say, refuses to acquiesce in the processes which he associates with 'maturity'. Richard, once his teacher and mentor and held in high esteem for his character and artistic ability, has now, as far as Vivaldo is concerned, sold out to the mediocrity of popular success – a mediocrity represented also by the figure of TV producer Ellis. Vivaldo (the name manages to suggest life – 'viva', music – Vivaldi, and a warm-blooded southern European ethnicity) becomes the vehicle for Baldwin's misanthropy. Looking out of his window, he sees a city full of people

> who got up in the morning and went to bed at night and, mainly, throughout their lives, to the same bed. They did whatever they were supposed to do . . . [they] were admirable because they were numerous. (pp. 104–5)

In the same scene, he imagines the sexual coupling which is proceeding in a flat opposite his building. Everything joyless, predictable, loveless and lustful, is here. In its awful coldness there is a repulsiveness reminiscent of Swift or of Samuel Beckett:

> Yes, he had been there: chafing and pushing and pounding, trying to awaken a frozen girl. The battle was awful because the girl wished to be awakened but was terrified of the unknown. Every movement that seemed to bring her closer to him, to bring them closer together, had its violent recoil, driving them farther apart. Both clung to a fantasy rather than to each other, tried to suck pleasure from the crannies of the mind, rather than surrender the secrets of the body. The tendrils of shame clutched at them, however they turned, all the dirty words they knew commented on all they did. These words sometimes brought on the climax – joylessly, with loathing, and too soon. The best that he had managed in bed, so far, had been the maximum of relief with the minimum of hostility. (p. 106)

Such people build such a city as New York. The indictment being laid is specifically against the urban horror. In the opening scene, the huge neon sign of a hotel represents, like the advertising hording in Scott Fitzgerald's *The Great Gatsby,* a vacuous culture. Simply, 'the weight of the city was murderous' (p. 6) and later, 'everything they passed was wretched' (p. 92). And in summer it is worse. The heat and the noise destroy 'nerves and sanity and private lives and love affairs.' Everyone is hostile. 'It was a city without oases, run entirely . . . for money; and its citizens seemed to have lost entirely any sense of their right to renew themselves.' Eric thus feels in danger 'of being forever banished from any real sense of himself' (p. 252)

The language is more modern, more obviously influenced by the existentialists, but the sentiments hark back to the Europe of the previous century and to the contempt of convention, and of the masses, found in the writings of Flaubert and Chekhov. Cass sums up what is clearly Baldwin's own view of the United States:

> Hope? No, I don't think there's any hope. We're too empty here. . . . This isn't a country at all, it's a collection of football players and Eagle Scouts. Cowards. We think we're happy. We're not. We're doomed. (p. 323)

It is in this context of a general malaise in United States urban culture that one locates the individuals of Baldwin's story.

There is a rooted tradition in fiction of characters' introspection, particularly in the matter of love. Baldwin in this respect (in detailed ways which will become apparent as our argument proceeds) closely resembles Marcel Proust and Laurence Durrell, both of whom devoted massive energies and considerable space to the exploration of the changing and complex webs of feeling that love involves. A reading of these and other authors, combined with personal experience, make it plain that love is ineffable. Writers committed to rendering its quiddity in words, will forever hover in its vicinity without ever nailing it down. No once-and-for-all account can be given.

A typical Proust or Durrell fictional situation of this kind entails someone who feels that underneath what appear to be sentiments of love there lurk dark passions of antagonism, but under these in turn there is 'really' an absolute commitment which, however, in its turn, is 'really' based on pure egoism rather than the imagined altruism of the individual. And so on, *ad infinitum.* We are all familiar with these various layers of analysis and meaning; they are the inevitable result of introspection and manifest themselves in comments such as 'I wonder whether I did really love him'. Baldwin adopts this deeply probing, and finally exasperating, search:

> He wished that he could rescue her, that it was within his power to rescue her and make her life less hard. But it was only love which could accomplish the miracle of making a life bearable – only love, and love itself mostly failed; and he had never loved her. He had used her to find out something about himself. And even this was not true. He had used her in the hope of avoiding a confrontation with himself which he had, nevertheless, and with a vengeance, been forced to endure. (p. 322)

The restlessness of the search, in Baldwin's writing, for some elusive, fundamental truth can be exhilerating, but it can also seem suspect. For the problem with this kind of rigorous scrutiny of feeling, in art, is that it is interminable: underneath one layer there is always another purportedly being the 'real' feeling or motivation. Nevertheless, Baldwin's writing is based on a belief in the validity of the layered model. He is committed to the view that the 'deeper' one probes into oneself, and of course into others, the more that is admitted, the more sophisticated and analytical are the processes of introspection and the observation of others, the more one will 'know' in some impliedly absolute sense, about individuals.

Most of the anguish recorded in *Another Country* is caused by love. We are presented, as in the typical Iris Murdoch novel, with a group of characters involved in pairings which share several Murdochian features: first, the love sustaining the pairings is painful and fragile; secondly, the pairings are almost laughably improbable – not so much taken separately, but considered together. Thus, we find the following configurations in *Another Country*. (I confine myself only to those involving physical sex, but even here the list is extensive):

Rufus–Eric (gay relationship, short-lived, Rufus less sexually interested).
Eric–Yves (idyllic gay relationship).
Eric–Cass (gay/straight; experimental for both; short-lived).
Eric–Vivaldo (gay/straight; experimental for both; one day).
Cass–Richard (boring marriage).
Ida–Vivaldo (straight, troubled, plagued by jealousy and lack of trust).
Ida–Ellis (Ida sleeps with Ellis for social/financial advancement).
Vivaldo–Jane (stormy rupture after racist remark by Jane).
Rufus–Leona (physical violence, ends in suicide and madness respectively).

Even from such a raw list one can already infer two themes: instability, and the enormous variety of sexual experience open to human beings if only they dare to brave conventions. Most, of course, do not. This latter fact – that people are trapped in a tiny segment of possible experience, namely legally contracted heterosexual monogamy – represents yet another difference between the 'multitude' and the individual characters. In this respect, like Genet, Baldwin is an existentialist; he believes that human beings can transcend the 'given', the customary and the conventional – indeed, they must do this – and 'find themselves' through individualistic, daring and dangerous ways. It is especially instructive that critics of Baldwin are most virulent when rejecting this challenge to break out of the straight/strait-jacket of narrow choice. Here is a typical critical response to the challenge:

> Since bisexuality is hardly a matter of free choice among men – it not representing a cultural norm – its presentation as a viable alternative to generally existing modes of social behaviour is hardly realistic. . . . The implication that Rufus' life might have been saved had Vivaldo made some sexual gesture towards him (Baldwin would say a 'loving' gesture) simply suggests an option not generally available in this culture and one therefore expressive of Baldwin's utterly private sense of values and little else.[2]

The first sentence claims as a principle of conduct precisely that which the existentialist most passionately detests – the idea that one *can* only do what is within the 'cultural norms' and the 'existing modes of social behaviour'. As I understand Gibson's argument, it is this: bisexuality is unconventional; therefore representing it as taking place is unrealistic; that is, behaviour which is unconventional and anti-normative does not occur.

The argument is self-evidently absurd, but worth spelling out for what it tells us about a certain sort of critical approach. First, Gibson has no concept of the existence of gay people who will, actually, do things which are unconventional in the teeth of the fact that they are unconventional. I have to stress here that I am not speaking ironically. It is quite common for people of considerable mental powers to simply not believe in palpable realities which they deplore. (Despite the daily evidence that the greatest threat of child abuse in all forms comes from heterosexual parents, especially heterosexual fathers, the very same newspapers which report these incidents still persist in associating homosexuality with child abuse.)

Secondly, one can detect here something equally absurd, although not made explicit, namely, the notion that cultural norms and conventions are, by reason of their having that status, worthy to be followed, or at any rate incontestably more worthy than anything 'unconventional'. Gibson also falsely assumes that a warm and loving touch must indicate something 'grosser' than mere touch; the idea that Vivaldo could touch Rufus warmly and lovingly without some genital consequence is alien and literally incomprehensible to him. He also makes it clear that 'sexual' and 'loving' are difficult to reconcile. Would he say as much about straight relationships?

Here is a second example of critical reaction on the theme of sexual choice. We are told by John Lash that Baldwin is writing from 'the inside of a daring new freedom of sexual choice. . . . *The reader never enters this province, of course* [my italics], but he may easily feel that he is catching glimpses of its glamour, and that he is gaining an initiation of sorts into its mystique.'[3] In the phrase, '*The reader never enters this province, of course*', one finds exactly the same denial of reality as in the first example. The phrase presumably means that all the readers are heterosexual. There is of course a more subtle, though equally offensive, interpretation: the writer affects to claim that the behaviour described would be unthinkable amongst the distinguished company of the readers of the academic work in question, even though knowing full well that there actually are gay readers whom he is by this method attempting to shame.

And what can be made of the reference to 'glamour'? Whatever one might want to call the experiences of Baldwin's men in the field of sexuality and personal relations – and those experiences are miraculous, tortured, exhilarating and destructive by turns – the very last word one would want to use in connection with them would be 'glamour', with its suggestion of the superficial and the meretricious. Similarly, 'initiation' and 'mystique' sound more like the Freemasons than the everyday love of man for man.

Baldwin describes love exhaustively, sometimes tediously, in order to describe feeling generally; what it is like to have emotions; the feeling of feeling. And the descriptions are not tidily discrete. Love is intimately linked to jealously, lust, ambition, failure, racism, hate. And the fragility of love is a constant theme. Thus, Eric and Yves appear for the first time having an idyllic time in France, by the sea; the scene is the exact opposite of the novel's opening depiction of the destitute Rufus. But they must break the enchantment and go – separately, hesitantly – to the States. The pretext is that Eric's career beckons, and there is validity in that reason. But beyond it there is a need for testing. How do I know you love me, if the going isn't tough? Always, there must be movement, doubt, the possibility of desertion. The relationships in the novel resemble Karl Popper's principle of falsifiability: if the pairing is not at least capable to dissolving, it can't be real enough, intense enough.

Lives experienced at this level of intensity are confusing. Baldwin makes readers share this confusion. For example, once Vivaldo has formed a relationship with Ida, he becomes exaggeratedly jealous over the possibility that she might be unfaithful with the unattractive but influential Ellis. As the signs of groundless and absurd jealousy mount, we become increasingly impatient with Vivaldo's lack of trust. How can he be so foolish? Then, it transpires she *has been* unfaithful. Baldwin has set us up, tricked us into a certainty of Ida's fidelity, only to disabuse us violently. To some extent, we are placed in Vivaldo's own position; our shock is his.

Or again, Leona loves Rufus passionately; and yet he beats her viciously, frequently. Is it because she is clinging to him as to a raft, that no one else would have her? Or that there is a strong masochistic (indeed suicidal) element in her character? Is she (in the psychoanalytic tradition) programmed by her unconscious to walk into destruction, or has she, in despair of the world, made an existentialist choice? Vivaldo tells her to leave Rufus; in reply she indirectly asserts a psychoanalytical point of view, namely that Rufus is a programmed inividual who 'can't help it': 'He wasn't like this when I met him, he's not really like this at all. I *know* he's not. Something's got all twisted up in his mind and he can't help it.' All these contradictions are summed up in her appearance: 'Her face was hideous, was unutterably beautiful with grief' (p. 49).

All desire is contradictory. In the opening scene, Rufus, utterly destitute, wants to be recognised by someone so that they can come to his aid; and yet in his shame he hopes the opposite, that he will pass unnoticed. Later, Rufus speaks to Vivaldo:

> 'Don't mind me. I know you're the only friend I've got left in the world, Vivaldo.'
>
> And that's why you hate me, Vivaldo thought, feeling still and helpless and sad. (p. 59)

What is especially impressive in Baldwin is that the reasons threatening the various relationships are never exhaustively spelt out; what we have instead is a general kind of background noise of urban decay, ageing, frustrated (Richard) or vaulting (Ida) ambitions, sexual experimentation (Vivaldo with Eric, Eric and Cass with each other), racism (Ida's and Rufus' 'revenge' on Whites through sex) and dishonesty. And they are often intertwined, and endlessly complex. For example, Ida reproaches Vivaldo: 'I used to hate you . . . for pretending to believe me [about her whereabouts when she was having an affair with Ellis] because you didn't want to know what was happening to me' (p. 335). But if so, why did she pretend to accept his pretence?

I shall now say something in greater detail about the male–male relationships. That between Eric and Rufus is perhaps the least easy to account for. Not only is Rufus shown as predominantly straight, but he is homophobic: 'perhaps he had allowed Eric to make love to him in order to despise him more completely' (p. 38). This is something of a conundrum: 'Rufus had despised him because he came from Alabama' (p. 38). Alabama, in the novel, is effectively made synonymous with racism; it is therefore a place where Rufus would be despised by White racists. Does he despise Eric because he comes from a racist state? Or perhaps he thinks of him as simply a country bumpkin, lacking urban sophistication? At any rate, their sexual relationship seems founded on negative and uncertain grounds.

Eric's own motives are questioned in the relationship with Rufus:

> But had he ever loved Rufus? Or had it simply been rage and nostalgia and guilt? and shame? Was it the body of Rufus to which he had clung, or the bodies of dark men, seen briefly, somewhere, in a garden, or a clearing, long ago, sweat running down their chocolate chests and shoulders, their voices ringing out, the white of their jock-straps beautiful against their skin. . . . Certainly he had never succeeeded in making Rufus believe he loved him. Perhaps Rufus had looked into his eyes and seen those dark men Eric saw, and hated him for it.
>
> (p. 155)

Sex is never merely itself. Rufus's suspicion of being 'used' – in this case as a kind of surrogate for a fantasy of (impliedly undifferentiated) black men – is, at root, everyone's suspicion in this book. They all want an answer to the question: 'does s/he *really* love me?' without realising that the word 'really' in this sentence has no semantic status. Baldwin himself hardly seems to realise this, which makes some of the descriptions of the anguishings, at least from this point of view, supererogatory.

Much more hopeful is the relationship between Eric and Vivaldo. The latter has hardly any sexual desire, but much love, for Eric. For one day, only, they make love. Afterwards, Vivaldo explains why the experience cannot be repeated:

> 'This day is almost over. How long will it be before such a day comes for us again? Because we're not kids, we know what life is like, and how time just vanishes, runs away – I can't, really, like from moment to moment, day to day, month to month, make you less lonely. Or you, me. We aren't driven in the same directions and I can't help that, any more than you can.' He paused, watching Eric with enormous, tormented eyes. He smiled. 'It would be wonderful if it could be like that; you're very beautiful, Eric. But I don't, really, dig you the way I guess you must dig me. You know? And if we tried to arrange it, prolong it, control it, if we tried to take more than what we've – by some miracle, some miracle, I swear – stumbled on, then I'd just become a parasite and we'd both shrivel. So what can we really do for each other except – just love each other and be each other's witness? And haven't we got the right to hope – for more? So that we can really stretch into whoever we really are? Don't you think so?' And, before Eric could answer, he took a large swallow of whisky and said in a different tone, a lower voice, 'Because, you know, when I was in the bathroom, I was thinking that, yes, I loved being in your arms, holding you' – he flushed and looked up into Eric's face again – 'why not, it's warm, I'm sensual, I like – you – the way you love me, but' – he looked down again – 'it's not my battle, not my *thing*, and I know it, and I can't give up my battle. If I do, I'll die and if I die' – and now he looked up at Eric with a rueful, juvenile grin – 'you won't love me any more. And I want you to love me all my life.' (p. 315)

I find passages such as this very moving, and partly because they so courageously sacrifice certain niceties and practices of literary decorum in order to get where they are going. What adverse criticism would label as the flaws in this passage – its sentimentality, its pretentious use of hippy argot ('So that we can really stretch into whoever we really are?'), its apparent straying into meaninglessness, above all its wishful thinking (the straight critic thinks: this is the ultimate, unrealisable desire of the gay man: to 'convert', that is, get into bed, the ultimately unattainable, the straight man) – are risks taken in order to express something powerful. However dimly, and against the weightiest of odds, it holds out possibilities of life and of love not recognised in the official culture of the West.

Genet had spelt out his renunciation of allegiance to official culture. Baldwin does the same, through Eric, with equal eloquence but a finer issue. Eric does not have recourse to malice, which is often Genet's sustenance; rather, his existentialism is more hopeful and positive. It is a process of thinking up his own standards; as a gay man, he must invent the world as he goes along. The following passage is, in Baldwin's work, of canonic importance:

> His life, passions, trials, loves, were, at worst, filth, and, at best, disease in the eyes of the world, and crimes in the eyes of his countrymen. There were no standards for him except those he could make for himself. There were no standards for him because he could not accept the definitions, the hideously mechanical jargon of the age. He saw no one around him worth his envy, did not believe in the vast, grey sleep which was called security, did not believe in the cures, panaceas, and slogans which afflicted the world he knew; and this meant that he had to create his standards and make up his definitions as he went along. It was up to him to find out who he was, and it was his necessity to do this, so far as the witch doctors of the time were concerned, alone. (p. 170)

Eric's relationship with Yves is idyllic. The portrayal of the Frenchman has a softness which has survived in him, despite the sordidness and lovelessness of his adolescence. The relationship between the lovers has been criticised as unrealistically blissful. Several points should be made about this. First, like the lovers in *Giovanni's Room,* they are happy because they are alone; it is at moments of greatest privacy that they enjoy each other the most. Literally, their physical isolation in the French house (like the 'room' of *Giovanni's Room*) makes felicity possible. Implied in this is the comment that gays cannot be at ease in public; that the parks, the restaurants, the bars, the very streets, are places where only straights may flaunt their affections. Predictably, critics have interpreted this compulsory exclusion from the public world as a voluntary act of hiding, brought on by shame and typical of gay people. (In exactly the same way, the history of women shows that, having been excluded from the world of work and confined to domestic roles, their continued exclusion from spheres of influence is based on their supposedly inherent desire for domesticity.)

Secondly, Western culture historically posits two loci – the town and the country – and builds round the one (the city) a tradition of vice and corruption, and around the other (the country) a pastoral myth of idyllic happiness in pleasurable penury. In literature, music and painting, this myth is potent: the shepherd with his pan-pipes watching his flock in high summer, versus the drunken Hogarthian rake up to his neck in gambling debts and sexual intrigues. It seems that such a binary opposition, between two utterly contrary modes, gives art of all genres much of its force. Baldwin makes use of this tradition, not by comparing city and country, but America and Europe. The distinction is not in fact as crude as the city/country dichotomy. But certain things are clear: there is a generosity, a human scale, a warmth and beauty about the experience of living in France (both in city and country) which is not found in his accounts of America. The latter is associated with pain, anguish, racism and urban ugliness. A comparison of the first page of Book One (p. 5) with the first page of Book Two (p. 147) illustrates the difference.

The France/United States contrast is largely based on Baldwin's own personal experiences of both places; it also has interesting echoes of Henry James's fictional contrasting of Europe and the United States. It works also on the metaphorical level. Baldwin wants to show that same-sex lovers can achieve personal fulfilment, that it is societies and cultures rather than innate individual human characteristics which put a stop to human flourishing. This point is not of course philosophically rigorous (societies are, in one sense, the creation of individuals, so the contrast is false) but it serves the artistic purpose of the book: the determination to present, in the teeth of the surrounding homophobic culture, a happy gay couple. Today, it would be called presenting 'positive images', and the antagonism towards it remains undiminished – as we can see from the British government's enacting of the notorious Clause 28 of the Local Government Bill 1988, attempting to suppress exactly those positive images.

Haunting Eric's present moments is the memory of his Alabama childhood; in that culture of puritanical values and racial prejudice, the sexual desire he felt for his black friend, LeRoy, is doomed from the start. The intricacies of how this relationship is socially perceived are spelt out; note, for example, that LeRoy is more 'knowing' about public opinion than Eric, for the oppressed are always forced away from naivety into a sort of worldliness by virtue of their situation. Only the privileged have access to innocence:

> . . . now their friendship, their effort to continue an impossible connection, was beginning to be a burden for them both. It would have been simpler – perhaps – if LeRoy had worked for Eric's family. Then all would have been permitted, would have been covered by the assumption of Eric's responsibility for his coloured boy. But, as things were, it was suspect, it was indecent, that a white boy, especially of Eric's class and difficult reputation, should 'run', as Eric incontestably did, after one of his inferiors. Eric had no choice but to run, to insist – LeRoy could certainly not come visiting him.
>
> And yet there was something absolutely humiliating in his position; he felt it very sharply and sadly, and he knew that LeRoy felt it too. Eric did not know, or perhaps he did not want to know, that he made LeRoy's life more difficult and increased the danger in which LeRoy walked – for LeRoy was considered 'bad', as lacking, that is, in respect for white people. Eric did not know, though of course LeRoy did, what was already being suggested about him all over town. Eric had not guessed, though LeRoy knew only too well, that the Negroes did not like him, either. They suspected the motives of his friendliness. They looked for the base one and naturally they found it. (p. 162)

In a crucial scene, the two friends are walking out together and of course they are alone, for they do not fit into any conceivably acceptable social pattern. Eric puts his arm around the other's shoulder and rubs the top of his head against LeRoy's chin. LeRoy puts his hand on Eric's neck. (By this we know something unpleasant is to come; for Baldwin's fiction trains us to expect enchantment to be followed by the smashing of dreams. We see it with Rufus's relationship with Leona, so apparently promising to start with, Cass with Richard, Vivaldo with Jane, Ida with Vivaldo, and so on; it is even, I believe, hinted at in Eric's relationship with Yves – 'even', because it is in this relationship that Baldwin, rather like Forster before him in *Maurice,* is insisting, against the probabilities, that two men can love and make each other happy on a long-term basis.)

The boys are confronted by the 'enemy'. Six young white people in a car rush past them – symbolically, dividing them from each other as the car passes between (reminding us of the end of Forster's *Passage to India,* where the two male friends' horses are sundered, as though deliberately, by the rocks) – and ridicule the boys' friendship by playing the tune of the wedding march on the car horn. LeRoy ironically draws the brutal moral: ' . . . *that's* where you supposed to be. You *ain't* supposed to be walking around this damn country with no nigger.' Eric is defiant in response, but unconvincingly so: '"I don't give a damn about those people," Eric said – but he knew that he was lying and he knew that LeRoy knew it, too . . .' (p. 163).

Baldwin's achievement, in this and many other episodes, is combining the themes of racism and homophobia. For, just as LeRoy's form of humiliation was universal for all blacks in the Alabama of the period, so the humiliation of having one's love ridiculed and driven wholly or partly underground, was and is universal for lesbians and gay men. The aching desire to love continues to do battle with the often incompatible but nevertheless powerful hope of integrating into society. On racial and sexual levels, this still goes on, and society often wins the battle. The result is individual treachery, acts of 'bad faith'. Natural allies side with the forces of the majority out of fear, and out of a desire to conform. They surrender their freedom and dignity and in return they receive, not a place in the sun, but a place in that dark hole-in-the-corner place which is the subject of Arthur Miller's plays.[4] Baldwin has the courage to say this, to refuse crude partisanship and tell the difficult truth.

Part of Baldwin's truth is that suffering oppression does not make one humane or tolerant. Rather the reverse. Of course, this has in the last ten years become a truism and a cliche, especially since Gore Vidal's influential essay, *Pink Triangle and Yellow Star*.[5] Vidal and others have pointed to the fanatical homophobic hatred of extreme American Jews; the anti-gay stance of Thatcher's Jewish cabinet ministers; the brutality of the Israeli government, and so on, drawing the conclusion that suffering does not inculcate sympathy for suffering, but rather makes one more likely to be an oppressor in similar fanatical vein. The most sensational British example of this occurred in 1988, when the British Chief Rabbi, Emmanuel Jacobowitz, called for the wholesale arrest of the entire non-celibate gay community; this despite his personal knowledge of Nazi concentration camps where gays were held together with his fellow Jews; shortly after his statement, which was widely reported, he became the only rabbi ever to be elevated to the House of Lords. Baldwin himself was repeatedly denounced and vilified – most famously by Eldridge Cleaver – because his sexuality was somehow thought to 'taint' the fight against racism.[6]

This terrible truth – terrible, and yet somehow exhilerating, for it demolishes a whole sentimental and mendacious tradition – does not of course apply only as between racial groups and gays.[7] However, as a member of both the groups in question, it is not difficult to see why Baldwin chose to concentrate his efforts here. We can compare him in this respect with Martin Sherman. As a gay man and a Jew, Sherman, in his astonishing play *Bent*, (based on authentic first-person accounts such as *The Men with the Pink Triangle* by Heinz Heger)[8] shows how, even in the Nazi concentration camps, Jewish prisoners were discriminating against gay inmates and humiliating them. In British prisons, it is notorious that the most odious offenders (murderers and violent robbers) are morally outraged at the presence in the prison of gay men who, therefore, have to be isolated under Prison Rule 43.

The 'why' of this syndrome is not difficult to find. As in Molière's *L'Avare*, the master hits the cook, so the cook hits the lower servant, in order to feel better. This hierarchy of contempt keeps a kind of psychic order and works well except for those at the bottom: gay people. They can, of course, and do, turn on others in their turn, but not with conviction. The black who shouts 'faggot' has more conviction than the gay who shouts 'nigger'; society accepts the hierarchical ordering implicit in the first but not the second. (One notes in passing, therefore, that in popular culture – for example, Hollywood films and ethnic magazines – we often see the first but nothing of the second.)

There are examples of this in *Another Country*. An Italian youth, in the park, looks with hate at the white/black pair of Leona and Rufus. Rufus replies with the single word 'Faggot' (p. 26). Like a witty repartee which surprises one's haughty interlocutor, the reply is seen as 'winning' the exchange for Rufus. Simply, homophobic put-downs supercede racist ones. Rufus's sister, Ida, the lifelong and embittered victim of racist attitudes and actions, also despises gays. She describes Eric as 'some poor-white faggot from Alabama' (p. 257) and as 'sick' (p. 258).

Vivaldo describes how one of the results of his tough and poor urban upbringing was (as it is, even more so, in today's society) a schooling in gay-bashing. You learn to hate from the teachers and the priests; then you *do* it:

> 'One time,' he said, 'we got into a car and drove over to the Village and we picked up this queer, a young guy, and we drove him back to Brooklyn. Poor guy, he was scared green before we got him halfway there but he couldn't jump out of the car. We drove into this garage, there were seven of us, and we made him go down on all of us and then we beat the piss out of him and took all his money and took his clothes and left him lying on the cement floor, and, you know, it was winter. . . . Sometimes I still wonder if they found him in time, or if he died, or what. (p. 91)

In this society, you cannot be left to yourself. You have to take part in the collective vandalism: 'You had to be a man where I come from, and you had to prove it, prove it all the time' (p. 90). This means attacking those who are not 'men'. Baldwin sees that the attacker suffers with his victim, for in the above episode, it is Vivaldo's humiliation – to have been a consenting part of such a mob – which exists side by side with that of the more obvious victim. In systems of oppression, all are losers.

Being ostracised and physically attacked for being gay is painful; but what makes Baldwin's account of gayness avoid the darkly pessimistic is that there are, too, significant gains. The outsider often sees through the nightmare of conformity, and is thereby able to avoid its soporific blandishments.

Ida reacts against her brother's white girlfriend:

> You'd never even have looked at that girl, Rufus, if she'd been black. But you'll pick up any white trash just because she's white. What's the matter – you ashamed of being black?
> (pp. 24–5)

Is Ida's use of 'white trash' retaliatory, a sort of counter-racism? Or is it a prejudice she takes for granted and is hardly aware of, so that she doesn't 'hear' it? Or is it merely descriptive, with no intended or sublimated derogatory connotation? Questions of this kind, and the subtle echoes of them, are the very stuff of Baldwin's musing on prejudice of all kinds. He wants to insist, for example, that most people are passive victims of prejudice, which exists as part of the difficult-to-change state of affairs; it seems 'natural', having what Roland Barthes called the 'taken-for-grantedness of the status quo'. There is very little implied sense of the possibilities of dislodging prejudice through political action or revolution. The pathetic figure of Leona, repeatedly beaten up by Rufus in what is, *inter alia*, a sort of racial revenge, is described by the narrator as the 'unwitting heiress of generations of bitterness' (p. 50)

The race issue in Baldwin gives rise to two typical situations. The first is that the black person, habituated throughout her/his life to hostility, anticipates it, expects it, steels her/himself to it – this, of course, is not a state of mind conducive to socialising with those who do not, as it turns out, display prejudice. Frequently, the result is moroseness and suspicion. In the bars and sidewalks of Baldwin's New York, no black person can ever really relax. Again, the modern gay parallel is close: when we walk down the street as a couple, or kiss, this is always a political and consciously public act. In a curious way, homophobes are right to say that it is a display – in this limited respect, that we know that it can, and very frequently it does, lead to hostility, verbal abuse and physical attack. The tension is always there. The 'innocent' or 'private' kiss in public is simply not available to us.

The second typical situation is the white impatience with this suspicion. When Vivaldo and Eric are talking about their love for, respectively, Ida and Rufus, Vivaldo complains that Ida never lets him forget her colour. She uses it as a weapon and a reproach, obsessionally. He asks: 'did Rufus do that to you. Did he try to make you pay?' Eric replies: 'Ah. He didn't *try*. I paid.' (p. 271). The point is summed up at the end of the novel by Vivaldo's dismissive comment to Ida: 'You want to hate me because I'm white, because it's easier for you that way' (p. 329). I take this to mean: 'with deliberate, or half-deliberate dishonesty, you blame racism when you can't face the real issue, which might be connected partly or wholly with your own personal inadequacies'. Once again Baldwin's painful probing of motives rises above crude partisanship; it is little wonder he was rejected by many in the macho circles of Black Power.

The emotional configurations arising from race issues sometimes lead in Baldwin to a manic introspection in the characters which is simply self-indulgent or bizarre. For example, he seems to attribute moral blame to unconscious racist impulses; whereas it is generally held that blame can only be associated with free choice or, to put it in the philosophers' phrase, 'ought implies can'. Thus Vivaldo:

> And he thought, very unwillingly, that perhaps he did not love her. Perhaps it was only because she was not white that he dared to bring her the offering of himself. Perhaps he had felt, somewhere, at the very bottom of himself, that she would not dare to despise him. (p. 236)

What we remember above all about Baldwin's writing on race in this novel is the rare combination of passion and intellectual distinction. Vivaldo and Cass are talking about the dead Rufus. Vivaldo says: 'They're coloured and I'm white but the same things have happened, really the *same* things, and how can I make them know that?' Cass tells him: 'But they didn't happen to you *because* you were white' (p. 92). Baldwin realised that non-blacks, non-gays, literally *do not know* things of this kind. And therefore they have to be told. When Flannery O'Connor was asked why her short stories were so violent and melodramatic, appearing as it were to ram their messages down the throats of her public, she simply pointed out that for those who were deaf it was necessary to shout. Baldwin, in this respect, shouts at the top of his lungs.

* * *

Another Country was published in 1962, *Giovanni's Room* in 1956. The distance Baldwin travelled in those six years can be measured by comparing the two works. The earlier novel has, in embryo, some of the qualities of the later masterpiece, but it is vitiated by a lack of courage. Baldwin had not yet opened out to see the interconnectedness of things, which is the quality, above all, informing *Another Country*.

Baldwin usually cannot bring himself to accept the validity of gay relationships on their own terms; they must be cast in the mould of straight relationships. Specifically, they must share the culture of buddy-machismo. This is particularly true throughout *Giovanni's Room*, but even in *Another Country*, the relationship of Rufus and Eric is like this:

> They were friends, far beyond the reach of anything so banal and corny as colour. They had slept together, got drunk together, balled chicks together, cursed each other out, and loaned each other money. (p. 107)

This is the equivalent of the buddy film/television series scenario (*Starsky and Hutch* and a thousand others going back to the interracial male pairings in Fenimore Cooper and Mark Twain). Notice that straight men are incapable of expressing affection for each other except through insult; that is the meaning of 'cursed each other out'. It does not just mean: they had a stormy relationship which weathered even bad arguments; it also means: a certain kind of verbal aggressiveness is itself a sign of affection. In armies, collieries and other male communities living dangerously or at high tension, it is common to hear men, in moments of exceptional tenderness, tell the object of their love that they are bastards or shitheads. It is an apology for breaching the code which prohibits such affection; it is the way they show they are not queers.

In this tradition, women are marginalised: seducing/fucking them is a thing the men do, as it were, *together*; women are 'chicks' (that is, lacking human status, inconsequencial, 'dumb', consumer objects, immature) and the activity of 'balling' them is equivalent to getting drunk or lending each other money. It is no big deal. The solidarity is between the men; there is no conceivable sense of solidarity with the women. The women have to be there, however (in the television series, the cops' girlfriends are glimpsed once every month or two for perhaps a minute), as a guarantee of the heterosexuality of the men. This tradition which exists amongst straight men is frequently taken over by gay men as a disguise; it allows them to express their desire for other men under the cloak of a straight tradition, and unfortunately Baldwin frequently employs this tradition in *Giovanni's Room.*

One of its components is a special, and especially repellant, kind of homophobia of which Baldwin is guilty time and again. (He was guilty of this in his life as well as his books.) It's essence is this: 'there are ordinary virile men who just happen to desire other men but are in all other respects entirely "normal"; then there are disgusting, effeminate fairies'. This brand of homophobia is unique to gay men (straights do not thus distinguish) and when voiced is meant as a plea to the straight majority, based on a rejection of the effeminate. The 'straight-acting' gay man (this term can still be seen in contact ads) asks for acceptance from straight society, and the price that he thinks might be sufficient for this (of course it never is) is betrayal of his fellows. In effect, he says: 'I am not like *them* I am just like you. My being like you is proved by my hating *them*'.

Consider this passage:

> They moved about the bar incessantly, cadging cigarettes and drinks, with something behind their eyes at once terribly vulnerable and terribly hard. They were, of course, *les folles,* always dressed in the most improbable combinations, screaming like parrots the details of their latest love-affairs – their love-affairs always seemed to be hilarious. Occasionally one would swoop in, quite late in the evening, to convey the news that he – but they always called each other 'she' – had just spent time with a celebrated movie star, or boxer. Then all of the others closed in on this newcomer and they looked like a peacock garden and sounded like a barnyard. I always found it difficult to believe that they ever went to bed with anybody[,] for a man who wanted a woman would certainly have rather had a real one and a man who wanted a man would certainly not want one of *them.* (p. 30)

Or this:

> He asked me if we were living together. I think perhaps I should have lied to him but I did not see any reason to lie to such a disgusting old fairy, so I said *Bien sûr*. . . . I began to get sick watching him and listening to him. (p. 102)

This becomes a kind of refrain: 'your disgusting band of fairies' (p. 132); 'he was just a disgusting old fairy' (p. 142). Ageism is often part of this: 'the least these dirty old men could do was *pay*' (p. 50).

The central dilemma at the heart of the novel is David's bisexuality. On the one hand he sees the value, and feels the love, of the beautiful Giovanni; on the other, he longs for the settled, sedate commitment to marriage represented by Hella. The novel is a record of his oscillating between these two, and sometimes taking comfort elsewhere (the one-night stand with the sailor). However, the novel lacks the coherence of *Another Country* because whilst purporting to be about bisexual anguish, it often appears to be about the anguish of a gay novelist indirectly 'coming out' through the thoughts and deeds of the (? intendedly sympathetic) character of David. Traditionally in the gay community, the declaration of bisexual desire was often seen as a half-way house; someone cannot face a complete 'coming out' and adopts this compromise to test the water. The raw desperate poetry of key passages in *Another Country*, impressive because devastatingly honest, is absent here. The author is not honest, and the anguish sounds self-indulgent and false:

> Perhaps, as we say in America, I wanted to find myself. This is an interesting phrase, not current as far as I know in the language of any other people, which certainly does not mean what it says but betrays a nagging suspicion that something has been misplaced. I think now that if I had had any intimation that the self I was going to find would turn out to be only the same self from which I had spent so much time in flight, I would have stayed at home. But again, I think I knew, at the very bottom of my heart, exactly what I was doing when I took the boat for France. (p. 25)

The strengths of *Giovanni's Room* reside in those features which are to appear most fully developed in *Another Country*. The first is Baldwin's refusal to allow us a cosy view of love; even when a relationship appears most perfect, it can always be shown to exhibit incipient decay: 'Nobody can stay in the Garden of Eden' (p. 28). (Compare this to the introduction of the Eric–Yves relationship in *Another Country*, in the Eden of the South of France, and the immediate threat to their happy complacency.) At the beginning of Part II we are told:

> In the beginning our life together held a joy and amazement which was newborn every day. Beneath the joy, of course, was anguish and beneath the amazement was fear. . . .' (p. 73)

Of course. No moment is so innocent that it cannot be tainted by reflection, no state of mind so serene that it is not vulnerable to the nudging in of despair:

> We had bought a kilo of cherries and we were eating them as we walked along. We were both insufferably childish and high-spirited that afternoon and the spectacle we presented, two grown men, jostling each other on the wide sidewalk, and aiming the cherry-pips, as though they were spitballs, into each other's faces, must have been outrageous. And I realised that such childishness was fantastic at my age and the happiness out of which it sprang yet more so; for that moment I really loved Giovanni, who had never seemed more beautiful than he was that afternoon. . . . Yet, at that very moment, there passed between us on the pavement another boy, a stranger, and I invested him at once with Giovanni's beauty. . . . I felt sorrow and shame and panic and great bitterness . . . one day I would not be with Giovanni any more. And would I then, like all the others, find myself turning and following all kinds of boys down God knows what dark avenues, into what dark places? . . . there opened in me a hatred for Giovanni which was as powerful as my love and which was nourished by the same roots. (pp. 80–1)

Like Genet and Williams, Baldwin always insists on love's fragility and transience. The novel's title has some relevance here, for 'the room' in its cramped awkwardness is a symbol of the sexual panic and claustrophobia suffered by David. Its being far from the centre, at Nation, signals what appears to David the peripheral experience of gay love. Giovanni has painted out the ground floor window and sits quite still next to it, in tension, when there are people to be heard on the other side of the window whom he cannot see – all of which is suggestive of gay closetry and secrecy. Giovanni's attempts literally to demolish part of the walls and build an alcove (that is, an extension) for books, is yet another (admittedly rather laboured) symbol of the need to break out of the relationship.

The second aspect of *Giovanni's Room* which anticipates *Another Country* is the skilful presentation of character, in which the idea of people being fixed in any set of dispositions or traits is eschewed. The often sympathetic David can be repellant: the early story of his betrayal of his love for Joey is echoed in different sorts of betrayal of Hella and Giovanni. He is the typical heartless deserter. He is irritatingly undirected in his life, constantly vacillating. Yet parts of his anguish manage to touch us. Giovanni often appears pathetically dependent and doomed, but at other times he is described as dangerous and threatening. Jacques is introduced kindly, but later becomes part of the stereotype of the old man hanging around glittering youth. Hella is represented as 'understanding' in the early stages, but by the time of the confrontation with David in the South of France, she is shrill and coarse.

This shifting of perspectives in relation to characters is mirrored by the nature of the episodes themselves. Rarely staying in the same emotional key, they move from gaiety to melancholy, from celebration to the funereal. A good example is the languid evening spent at the gay bar ('that gloomy tunnel' – p. 45) when David first meets Giovanni, which is immediately followed by the breakfast scene at Les Halles, which is good-humoured and full of a burgeoning sense of human possibilities.

Giovanni's Room is too embarrassed by the full implications of its subject matter. It enters bravely, but then shrinks away. It is, most significantly, informed by a collaborator's shame. But it is the beginning of the road which leads to one of the finest novels of our time.

10

The Plays of Joe Orton

Joe Orton (1933–67) was brought up, one of four children, in a working-class family in Leicester. His mother was a machinist and his father a gardener. There was little affection in the family, and Orton's lifelong hatred of tedious provincial life clearly owes much to his early years at home. He was not successful at school, although he did manage to learn shorthand and accounting at a business college. He had a variety of jobs between sixteen and eighteen, but he was sacked from all of them because, according to him, he resented having to go to work in the morning. Theatre offered an escape from boredom, and he got into RADA, where he met his future lover, Kenneth Halliwell. The latter, seven years older than his partner, was academically bright and introduced Orton to vast tracts of literature entirely new to the younger man. Both of them began to write together a series of novels (heavily influenced by Ronald Firbank) which were not published. After 1957, they wrote separately. In 1962 both of them were imprisoned for defacing library books; Orton admitted that it was probably true that one of the reasons for doing this was resentment at lack of literary success. Suddenly, with Entertaining Mr Sloane *(1964) Orton – who was obsessed with the need for fame and recognition – struck lucky. The next few years were to see more plays accepted, a commission from the Beatles for a screenplay, trips to Morocco for the Arab boys. Halliwell, who was in any case extremely unstable, couldn't take the pressure of Orton's growing success and his resulting jealousy and resentment. On 10 August 1967, in one of the most famous British murders of the century, he battered Orton to death with a hammer and then took his own life with an overdose of pills. Orton left behind him a series of diaries (sexually frank and often hilarious), which are now published.*

The literary criticism of Orton's work is insistently based on the biographical. This is largely because of the exciting nature of many of the events in his life, which culminated in his sensational murder by his lover Kenneth Halliwell. The way in which Orton lived his life has occupied a central place in the commentaries, most notably that by John Lahr.[1] Orton's outlandishness, the freshness of his rage, the immaturity of his acts of bravado (such as defacing hundreds of library books in the Islington Public Library, for which he was sent to prison), and the extent of his promiscuity – all these details have been requisitioned by critics as yet more evidence of the 'true' nature of homosexuality. The Orton story, like the advent of AIDS in the early 1980s, presented the establishment with a unmissable opportunity to reinforce homophobic mythology: gay men as 'outrageous' (often a code word for 'gay'), hostile to women, over-concerned with sex, with a clever wit and few moral principles.

The way in which Orton's life and work has spawned a whole crew of directors, professors and assorted media commentators who have contributed to this – and in the process been prepared to censor or change the text of the plays so that they fit more conveniently into their own preferred ideas – is an intriguing story. I do not propose to tell it myself, because I have been forestalled by an excellent study which does just this, written by Simon Shepherd.[2] This is the best book on Orton, and contains a sustained and detailed account of how heterosexist assumptions govern literary interpretation, and those genuinely interested in Orton should read it.

Shepherd's weakness is in overestimating the plays themselves. Essentially they are farces with a serious purpose. Orton made it clear that he wanted his satirical points to hit home with terrific force. His hatred of the establishment, and his placing it in the line of fire, is not disputed. But in my view the enterprise doesn't come off. This is because it is based on the premise that audiences will take the serious points to heart. Clearly, this is hardly ever the case. On at least a dozen occasions in the past twelve years I have sat in the National Theatre or the RSC and seen a radical play attacking all the bourgeois values held by those very people sitting in the theatre – and those people have lapped it up, secure in the knowledge that it is *their* world, and all that radical authors can do is to gently rock the boat a little from time to time.

If one looks at contemporaneous reactions to the Orton farces in the newspaper reviews, one sees that they clearly divide into two groups: the more adventurous are wonderfully amused; the more staid talk of filth and censorship. Rarely do the reviews discuss the attack on British society which for Orton was their main thrust. He blamed the productions for not having the desired effect: 'The play [*Ruffian on the Stair*] is not written naturalistically, but it must be directed and acted with absolute realism. . . . No "stylization", no "camp" . . .' and of another play he said, '"Loot" is a serious play . . . Unless "Loot" is directed and acted perfectly seriously the play will fail. . . . A director who imagines that the only object is to get a laugh is not for me.[3]

Despite Orton's desire not to see his plays produced with 'camp' acting, very many of the scenes and individual lines are the very essence of 'camp'; namely, exaggerated comic action combined with verbal wit whose joint effect is to invite us to face bravely a world which, not looked at thus awry, would seem too awful. In some of the plays, especially *Ruffian on the Stair* and *The Erpingham Camp,* we see the prankery which prompted Orton to deface the library books, and the quality of the humour (on the surface, feeble and over extended) is reminiscent of the library escapade:

> ERPINGHAM. Is number four latrine unblocked?
> RILEY. Yes.
> ERPINGHAM. And the toddlers' paddling pool? Have you removed whatever was causing the disturbance?
> RILEY. Yes.
> ERPINGHAM. Good. What was it?
> RILEY. Two ducks. Made of plastic. They were stuck together.
> ERPINGHAM. Beak to beak? [*Pause*] Was the joinery smutty?
> RILEY. Well, sir – the Engineer in charge had to perform surgery.
> ERPINGHAM. Did the kiddies see?
> RILEY. No. They were having a quick run round with Matron.
> ERPINGHAM. I want those ducks destroyed. We've no time for hedonists here. My camp is a pure camp.[4]

The point, of course, is the ridiculing of prudery, and the mental banality of fascistic authoritarianism. There is skill, too, in the details; the simple use of 'kiddies' calls up a world of working-class sentimentality.

It is precisely the childish, blatant aspect of Orton's camp style – the aspect most likely to be criticised – which is its point. Orton has no intention of accepting the view that the sabotaging of the English culture in which he lives, and which he so detests, has to be conducted on enemy terms. Forster, Leavitt, Isherwood and Williams might be prepared to argue against prevailing norms, employing (for the most part) the urbane discourse of the opposition; Orton, by contrast, is an iconoclast. The novelty of introducing the most banal aspects of lavatory humour into theatre is triply shocking: first, because such humour is thought to be out of place in serious dramatic work; second, because, on the surface level of its Chaucerian bawdy, we are actually being invited to enjoy its raw appeal (as Orton himself surely does), and third because the coarseness is placed in the mouths of those characters representing the camp authorities (who stand, in some measure, for civic authority generally), and these characters hereby stand exposed as vulgarians in the widest sense. This kind of humour also allows Orton to introduce, directly or suggestively, the theme of homosexuality under the cover of the various *doubles entendre.*

This use of the farce format in order to make telling criticisms of society has other aspects. Chaos, both linguistic and situational, reigns in the world of farce; the unexpected, the improbable and the outlandish are the stuff of which it is made. Writing at the same time as the absurdist dramatists (Ionesco, Beckett, Pinter), Orton arrives at similar conclusions by a different route. The world is inexplicable and meaningless; its events are random; its rulers appear to take themselves seriously and to stand on their dignity whilst engaging in actions and words clearly risible to onlookers, who in turn are frequently too timid to point all this out.

Notoriously, the plays owe a great deal to the influence of Pinter. The terseness, pregnancy of phrase, inscrutablility, underlying absurdity, surface farce – all these come from Pinter. Take this, for example, from *Ruffian on the Stairs*:

WILSON [*smiling*]. I've come about the room.
JOYCE. I'm afraid there's been a mistake. I've nothing to do with allotting rooms. Make your enquiries elsewhere.

WILSON. I'm not coloured. I was brought up in the Home Counties.[5]

Less frequently, we get clear echoes of Oscar Wilde: witty

repartee combining linguistic facility with (implied) perceptive social comment:

> CAULFIELD. . . . Take a tip from a member of the criminal classes.
>
> MCCORQUODALE. All classes are criminal today. We live in an age of equality.[6]

> CAULFIELD. He's a defrocked priest. He made no secret of the fact that your wife was his only source of pleasure.
>
> PRINGLE. What a disgraceful admission. He ought to be put in prison and visited by myself.[7]

At its most successful, Orton's wit manages to combine a whole series of social observations and criticisms:

> MIKE. I'll maybe forgive her. Our Lord forgave the woman taken in adultery. But the circumstances were different. [*Pause*] It's a ludicrous business. Ludicrous. The deceit. At her age. She wants somebody younger. At her age they get the itch. It's like a tale told by a commercial traveller. Just for a few minutes' thrill. I don't know what she'd be like if we had a television.[8]

The smugness of the first sentence is upset by the awkward (that is, working class) placing of 'maybe'. (Orton, for all his proletarian roots, is forever laughing at the stuttering verbal infelicities of working class speech. Like Genet, his radicalism is anarchic and nothing to do with socialism's questionable elevation of the supposed dignity of the 'worker'.) The next two sentences give us an audacious reference to Christ. It is audacious not only because offensive to Christians who will hardly want to hear their leader referred to in the context of a farce, but also because of the sudden juxtaposition with what preceded it. The words 'It's a ludicrous business. Ludicrous. The deceit. At her age. She wants somebody younger' illustrate the staccato speech, and the repetitions, of the intellectually undistinguished. The well-observed use of 'they' ('they get the itch') shows us that Mike is the sort of man to sum up all women in this dismissive way. Because of the effect so far of a mindless speaker – most of the speech, as if to stress this, is a whole series of clichés and hackneyed phrases just glued together without thought – the introduction of the reference to *Macbeth* is all the more amusing.[9] The whole speech concludes with a final line which makes fun of the prophets of cultural doom who constantly identify modernity – represented here by television – as wicked. The quick-fire, dense hilarity of all this has the desired effect of making an inflated speaker appear pompous and absurd.

This 'density' often approaches the nature of one-liners given to an audience by stand-up comics: 'If my wife is committing adultery my position would be intolerable. Being completely without sin myself I'd have to cast the first stone. And I'm dead against violence'.[10] The use of biblical borrowings and clichés shows that the morality of the speaker is an unthinking one, involving the repetition of received 'positions', rather than a genuine engagement with human dilemmas. The most important basis for any moral system – the realisation that sets of precepts are in themselves never sufficient, as they often clash and then what is needed is a method of deciding between conflicting principles – is clearly absent from the character's attitude here. All we have is a set of grim imperatives picked up through socialisation in an arid and meaningless culture. Orton makes a similar point about the inadequacies of pre-packed moral systems in *The Erpingham Camp*, when Kenny says that he can't stand intolerant people and wants to beat them up.

Orton's wit should be considered in relation to two other features of his art: the outrageousness of the action itself, on the stage, and the implications for language of his immensely varied and dizzying use of words. An example of outrageousness opens *Ruffian on the Stair*:

> JOYCE. Have you got an appointment today?
> MIKE. Yes. I'm to be at King's Cross station at eleven. I'm meeting a man in the toilet.[11]

The word 'appointment' sounds like something connected with business, so that when we hear the location, we struggle with the choice of two interpretations: either that there is a business meeting taking place, with farcical improbability, in a public lavatory, or there is a sexual rendezvous, with the word 'appointment' being employed with comic inappropriateness.

(Pinter's dialogue is full of examples of mundane facts dressed up in dignified nouns like 'appointment'; and Orton's characters frequently try to bolster the importance of their lives and activities using the same device.) The point is that Orton can get away with a reference to a homosexual rendezvous in a public lavatory because the words conceivably bear an innocent interpretation as well. This, of course, is the music hall tradition of the *double entendre.* Hugely puritanical British and United States television audiences will allow comedy shows with the most extraordinary coarseness and obscenity provided there is the fig leaf of the secondary meaning. It is a paradigm of hypocrisy, an institutionalising of deceit.

A good example of this hypocrisy in action, ironically enough, is the title of Lahr's book, *Prick Up Your Ears*. Despite the obvious nature of the ears/arse anagram, the title is bandied about freely; it is extremely unlikely, however, that a title like *Prick Up Your Arse* would be countenanced on the front of a dust jacket.

A great many of Orton's jokes are *doubles entendres* of this kind. In one way, the manner in which they are presented, they conform to the strict conventions within which such coarseness is permitted. In another way, however, they are quite daring, because the subject matter is not (or not merely) smutty prurience, but the introduction of the taboo subject of homosexuality, which Orton hereby smuggles into his texts. Here is a classic case from *What the Butler Saw*. Dr Prentice has just told Nick to strip and he 'stares in admiration' at Nick's body as he says: 'Remarkable. My last secretary couldn't better you. And she was a descendant of Houdini.'[12] What is really going on – physical admiration – is 'covered' by the supposed subject matter, which is freeing oneself rapidly of clothes like an escapologist.

Orton's outrageousness – the dead body on stage in *Loot*, the gay incest of *Ruffian*, the sexual sharing of Sloane at the end of *Entertaining Mister Sloane*, the hoisting aloft (in the original version) of Churchill's penis in *What the Butler Saw* – arose from a spirit of anarchic defiance such as operates in the writings of Genet. Orton hoped that his plays would be beneficially shocking, throwing complacent audiences into self-examination and social criticism but, as I have already suggested, this hope is vain. One of the chief themes of this book is that of social defiance. Because for me this is expressed most successfully in *The Good and Faithful Servant*, we shall now turn to it.

Orton's disgust at the fact that a supposedly enlightened twentieth-century Western state should base its parliamentary, legal, moral and social codes on what he felt to be the repressive and authoritarian edicts of Christianity is reflected in the choice of title. The phrase is taken from one of Christ's parables, that of the talents. A master leaves behind him three servants: to the first he gives ten talents, to the second five, and to the last one. On his return, the first two servants have doubled their alloted money through skilful investment, and the master calls them 'good and faithful servants'; but the third has hidden his one talent out of fear of failure. The master says to him:

> You wicked, lazy servant! You should have put my money on deposit with the bankers, so that when I returned I would have received it back with interest. Take the talent from him and give it to the one who has the ten talents. For everyone who has will be given more, and he will have an abundance. Whoever does not have, even what he has will be taken from him. And throw that worthless servant outside, into the darkness, where there will be weeping and gnashing of teeth.[13]

In Orton's play, a 'good and faithful servant' (the eponymous character Buchanan) works for the same company for the whole of his life, and on retirement is thrown onto the scrap heap with only a couple of junk items to commemorate this event. This corresponds to the 'weeping and gnashing of teeth' in Matthew's gospel. In this way, Orton manages to attack the work ethic and the capitalist system, along with the Christianity which is constantly used to justify it and prop it up. An important part of the point is that Buchanan is a foolish but willing tool of the capitalist system, taking over the bosses' value system when assessing his own worth. The bosses take the money and Buchanan, after decades of tedious labour, is expected to be grateful for the pittance he has been receiving over the years. At the core of the play's meaning is the inability of Buchanan to see how and to what extent he has been exploited, and that his respect and awe for the company for which he has worked (and, by analogy, all the oppressive institutions and customs of society and the state) are radically misplaced.

The play opens with Buchanan arriving, after much searching, in the personnel section of the firm: 'I've found it at last. I've had a long journey.' Orton's point is that the firm is vast and impersonal: 'Didn't they provide a map?' the cleaner asks him.[14] Being thoroughly modern, the firm has of course put in place an apparatus which, superficially regarded, offers a warm, personal approach. There is a social club for ex-employees, and a welfare officer, Mrs Vealfoy, to offer advice on personal problems and to organise social events. The lifelessness of these arrangements is conveyed through Orton's sensitivity to the diction of 'officialese' and the vocabulary of the condescending social services. Showing Buchanan round the recreation centre, Mrs Vealfoy tells him:

> Over here we have dominoes, cards and darts and all the pastimes.
> [*She points out a group of* OLD MEN *and* WOMEN. *Two of them are in wheelchairs, one is blind, a couple are simple-minded. They stare at* BUCHANAN *without interest.* MRS VEALFOY *smiles and takes* BUCHANAN *across the room.*]
> And over here we have conversation. (pp. 183–4)

The single word 'pastimes' suggests something inoffensive, inert, safe, and shatteringly dull. And the notion that the members are so at a loss that 'conversation' has to be formally organised is an indictment not merely of a firm which has thus effectively turned them into robots, but an indictment of the workers who have acquiesced in the process.

At the heart of Buchanan's malaise is his acceptance of values that have been foisted upon him by institutions, so that he is nothing in himself apart from those props. In a dialogue with another pensioner, we see how both men have accorded importance to events which are actually trivial in the extreme:

> OLD MAN. Bowls is my sport.
> BUCHANAN. That's a nice game.
> OLD MAN. I was almost mentioned in a well-known sporting periodical once.
> BUCHANAN. I never got as far as that.
> OLD MAN. I regard that as the high-spot of my life.
> BUCHANAN. Yes. You would. [*Pause*] The high-spot of my own career came when my photo appeared in the magazine. I didn't ask them to put it in. Some of them go round canvassing for support in their claims to be included. But I

> stood aside. And one day they came to my department and insisted I pose for them. I was unwilling at first. But I realized it was for my own good. (p. 185)

A version of this last phrase is used by those in authority, in their attempts to cajole. Parents, teachers and bosses tell those in their power that certain measures are 'for your own good'. Buchanan's submission to authority is so complete that even the language he uses is that of those people which the play clearly presents as his natural enemies.

Earlier, Buchanan indicates indirectly to Mrs Vealfoy that he would like another photo taken of him to commemorate his retirement. This need to be recognised and validated by the firm shows not only a regrettable inability to devise his own standards, and his striving instead for the approval of an outside body, but it shows that people will choose even the most drastically inappropriate bodies as representatives of respectability and value.

Mrs Vealfoy's little farewell speech at Buchanan's retirement party is couched in the language of a public school yearbook: fake sentiments dressed in stuffy, semi-archaic clichés. Orton is brilliant at this sort of pastiche:

> George left school at fourteen and joined the firm one year later, receiving the princely sum of seven shillings a week – which he will tell you went a long way in those far-off times. He quickly became known for his speed and intolerance of any work which was in the least 'slip-shod'. . . . George has had his share of life's tragedies. We all remember reading that he was on the danger list some years ago. He soon returned to us, however, and his cheery laugh echoed once again through the canteen. He is now fit and still rides a bicycle. Nothing could quell George, I'm sure. (pp. 159–60)

In this play, Orton shows that people desperately need to cling to fixed ideas – however absurd or contradictory – and set social routines. Mrs Vealfoy asks Debbie if her parents would mind if she were to have an illegitimate baby. Debbie replies: 'Mum would die. She couldn't put it in the paper, see. She'd feel she'd been cheated' (p. 163). Later, Buchanan talks to Ray about the latter's future:

RAY. I don't work.

BUCHANAN. Not work! [*He stares, open-mouthed*] What do you do then?

RAY. I enjoy myself.

BUCHANAN. That's a terrible thing to do. I'm bowled over by this, I can tell you. It's my turn to be shocked now. You ought to have a steady job. (p. 167)

Buchanan has not learned his lesson. Despite his own disastrous life being tied to the wheel of labour – and the cost includes the loss of an arm, an injury sustained in the firm's service – he wants Ray to follow him. It may be, of course, that this is not stupidity but malice; his life has been ruined, so why should the younger generation escape?

Buchanan has lost all his individuality, a point marvellously illustrated in Scene 5, which has no dialogue and simply involves Buchanan removing his uniform and finally surrendering it. As he takes it off, it is placed piece by piece on a 'dummy', suggesting the mindlessness of all who wear such uniforms. Afterwards, he appears diminished. In his ordinary clothes, 'He appears smaller, shrunken and insignificant' (p. 164). And the end of Buchanan's life of work is marked by the presentation of an electric clock and a toaster. The clock represents the time, a lifetime, which Buchanan has sacrificed to the firm; the toaster, cheap and badly made, blows up when first plugged in:

RAY. Where did you get this load of old rubbish?

EDITH. Shhh! [*She nods to* BUCHANAN, *in a quiet voice to Ray*] It was presented to Mr Buchanan by his firm. As a reward for fifty years' service. (p. 168)

Towards the end of the play, Mrs Vealfoy wants to know why Buchanan appears to be brooding when, according to her, he should be jolly. She is the type of no-nonsense, pull-your-socks-up bully, exuding phoney intimacies ('May we be completely informal and call you George?' – p. 156) but possessing ruthlessness just below the surface ('Question him why he does that. Worm it out of him' – p. 179). We are being presented by Orton with a world of hardness, and this picture is reinforced in Edith's explanatory reply: 'Our grandson has misbehaved himself. The clock and the toaster have proved a disappointment. And to cap it all he's old. So what with one thing and another his attitude is of despair' (p. 179). There is a high comic talent here, in the bathos-in-reverse, and in combining an off-hand, matter-of-fact tone with terrible truths.

Buchanan's story is a vehicle for Orton's attack on the banality of modern life and the slavish attitudes of mind it encourages. The protagonist's life has been uneventful, valueless, passive. This point is anticipated early in the play when he is talking to Edith:

> BUCHANAN. You have philosophy then? [*EDITH nods, begins to scrub the floor*] Are you resigned to anything in particular?
> EDITH. No. Life in general. Isn't that enough? (p. 156)

Like Tennessee Williams, Orton's emphasis is on escape from drudgery, refusal of social orthodoxy, resistance to curbs on pleasure (in particular, sex) and rejection of all the lies necessary to build up a conformist society. Those lies are illustrated dramatically in this play through the use of cliché, symbolism (the dummy, the exploding toaster) and absurdity. *The Good and Faithful Servant* stands as a supremely effective attack on current Western values and as such may well come to supersede the more riotous farces in critical esteem.

11

Christopher Isherwood: *A Single Man*

Christopher Isherwood (1904–86) was born in Cheshire and educated at Repton School and at Cambridge. He studied medicine in London for one year before going to Berlin, where he taught English. Several novels resulted in this experience, such as Mr Norris Changes Trains *(1935) and* Goodbye to Berlin (1939). *In the 1930s, he collaborated with W. H. Auden on three plays. In 1938, he travelled with Auden to China, and published the first of his autobiographical works,* Lions and Shadows. *At the outbreak of world war, he went to the United States, where he lived until his death. He continued to write novels and autobiography, and became closely involved in the Vedanta Society of Los Angeles. In 1980 he published* My Guru and His Disciple, *the story of his friendship with, and tutelage under, the Swami Prabhavananda. For the latter part of his life he lived in an apparently stable and enriching relationship with Don Bachardy, an artist, in Santa Monica, California; both men became minor public symbols of 'the happy gay couple'. The warmth of that relationship is reflected in George's memory of his lover in* A Single Man.

In his novel, *A Single Man,*[1] Isherwood shows a man who 'came face to face with the lonely life of the ageing single man. . . . With devastating candour he strips away the protective skins of the lonely, frightened, homosexual, single man.' According, that is, to the blurb of the Penguin edition of 1969.[2] In fact, this blurb is entirely false,[3] and the reasons for its being so go far further than the usual explanations of bad or misleading blurbs (carelessness; crassness). What the novel does is to affirm the value and validity – indeed, the essential decency, if not actual superiority – of the gay hero, George. Reading it is an antidote to all those accounts of doomed and suicidal homosexuals which bespatter literary history, and which reinforce the ideology of the majority. An intelligent, detached observer of society, George's viewpoint is, more or less, the one we are invited to adopt as readers, as we are taken through a series of intelligible and reasonable political and personal attitudes: the belief in literature and art; the hatred of ugly modern landscapes; the hostility to students' insensitivity in the face of their studies; the materialism and petty bourgeois values of America; and so on.

Bearing in mind its date of first publication (1964), this is something new. Not only is there no sense at all of sexual guilt, or neurotic self-loathing, or suicidal tendencies – all the ingredients which the culture expects to find in a 'gay' novel, to confirm its mythology of homosexuality – the tables are turned and we are invited to see normative heterosexual family life, as represented by the Garfeins and the Strunks, as palid and vacuous. Gay values are taken for granted; they constitute the starting point; but heterosexuality is seen to threaten a life of tedious and innane conformity, in a sea of idiot and unlovely children.

This is not an acceptable message to convey; so the blurb 'changes' the message, or tries to. Two separate possibilities exist to explain the further meaning of this blurb. First, an intelligent blurb writer understands the novel's true message, but realises that only a deliberate misrepresentation of it will encourage browsers to buy the book – for that is the function of blurbs – since all browsers are, like blurb-writers, heterosexual. Secondly, and more likely, the novel's affirmative message is so obnoxious to the blurb writer that his/her mind simply does not allow the novel's meaning to register, in the same way that news of horrific events is often not accepted by the psyches of the affected persons, who 'refuse to believe it'.

I should say here that, in suggesting that the blurb writer has 'missed' or 'perverted' what I take to be obvious meanings in the novel, I appear to be undermining a well-established principle that no text has a fixed meaning, which will always depend on the varied responses which it elicits from different individuals, cultures and historical periods. Nevertheless, I am sympathetic to Nietzsche's position on knowledge, which is that although it can never be established with absolute certainty, certain accounts of states of affairs are more 'appropriate' (and therefore 'better') than others.

A Single Man is one of the earliest gay novels to shift the discussion of social pathology away from the oppressed group itself and onto the oppressing majority. It is a shift later mirrored in medical attitudes (always far behind intellectual currents) which in the 1970s began to analyse homophobia, rather than the supposed malfunctions of lesbians and gay men. Isherwood's analysis is bold, also, in the way in which he proceeds in this task: for the attack is launched not just on those heterosexuals whose homophobia is clearly a malignity resulting in all kinds of bigoted schemes and proposals; it is also launched against the nature and consequences of the *heterosexual life-style itself*, as it has developed in the particular conditions of an advanced Western capitalist society. I shall now describe both of these attacks.

The first can be illustrated from the narrator's treatment of Mr and Mrs Strunk. Mr Strunk is the one supposed to take the more extreme position:

> Mr Strunk, George supposes, tries to nail him down with a word. *Queer*, he doubtless growls. But, since this is after all the year nineteen sixty-two, even he may be expected to add, I don't give a damn what he does just as long as he stays away from me. Even psychologists disagree as to the conclusions which may be reached about the Mr Strunks of this world, on the basis of such a remark. The fact remains that Mr Strunk himself, to judge from the photograph of him taken in football uniform at college, used to be what many would call a living doll. (p. 20)

Points which are to emerge with greater frequency and force in succeeding years – so much so that they will become clichés – are here offered confidently. Mr Strunk's desire 'to nail him down with a word' suggests the whole psychodrama of prejudice, in which a complex personality is reduced and dehumanised by the imposition of a single mentally manageable concept. The growling suggests at the same time bad temper and a bestial connection. 'I don't give a damn . . .' is a parallel to the famous, 'some of my best friends are Jewish . . .', both based on the curious phenomenon that those most imbued with discriminatory tendencies are frequently those most certain within themselves that they are free of it. The phrase is also a cliché, so that Mr Strunk stands convicted, in readers' eyes, of the further offence of linguistic tiredness and of being intellectually facile. The passage then ends with a speculation about Mr Strunk, showing that there must surely be something 'wrong', even perhaps paranoid, about someone who allows himself to be so threatened by the fact of homosexuality. (This last point is, of course, something we have already seen in action in *Cat on a Hot Tin Roof*.) We are finally told, in a comically teasing apparent *non sequitur*, that Mr Strunk was 'a living doll' (that is, handsome) in his youth. Does this suggest actual homosexual experience for which he now wishes to atone through vehement moralism,[4] or an incipient gay desire ('doll' carries some of the passive, effeminate connotations favoured by heterosexuals when discussing gay men), the price of suppressing which is a vocal prejudice? (There are countless examples of this, especially in political and judicial life: anti-gay bigots by day, rent-boy lovers by night.)

Mrs Strunk, on the other hand, thinks of herself as a 'liberal', but what this involves for her is that gay sexuality as 'evil' has been displaced by gay sexuality as 'sick', which is hardly any improvement. It simply corresponds with the gradual replacement of religious or moral explanations with secular, 'scientific' ones:

> Some cases, caught young enough, *may* respond to therapy. As for the rest – ah, it's so sad; especially when it happens, as let's face it it does, to truly worthwhile people, people who might have had so much to offer. (Even when they are geniuses in spite of it, their masterpieces are invariably *warped*.) So let us be understanding, shall we, and remember that, after all, there *were* the Greeks (though that was a bit different, because they were pagans rather than neurotics). Let us even go so far as to say that this kind of relationship can sometimes be almost beautiful – particularly if one of the parties is already dead; or, better yet, both. (p. 20)

We are impressed by the accuracy of this (we have all heard Mrs Strunks with their self-satisfaction and undeserved sense of superiority) but also by the huge ironic gap between Mrs Strunk's assumption that her view is 'advanced', fair-minded and humane, and the reader's outrage at her intolerable and culpable blindness. Incidentally, the theme of the 'happy death' (= death is the best thing that could have happened), represented bitterly in the last sentence (Isherwood loses narrative control here; his anger makes him depart suddenly from free indirect style into the bitterly ironic) is mirrored in the coarse slogans of fascist graffiti. A frequently found one is 'The only happy homosexual is a dead one.'

Isherwood does not make the mistake of balancing this bigotry with an angelic or forgiving victim. George's response, at least occasionally (and especially in his car, when he feels he can indulge such feelings), is hate. He has a regular fantasy that he is a sinister and powerful figure of terror who can kill or torture all the bigots with utter ruthlessness, unless they agree to effect progressive social changes to end homophobic practices. A lust for killing develops, to purge his victimised status. Certainly, this inevitable feature of the psyches of the oppressed is as universal in individuals affected, as the knowledge of it is absent from either the consciousness or the media of the oppressors. Very few lesbians or gay men do not experience this hate; but equally, no heterosexual can really be brought to believe in it. Isherwood's avoidance of sentimentalising George's character – a danger, in view of his bereaved status – is of key importance; for readers who might weep over him would see him as pathetic (therefore weak and unempowered, therefore essentially contemptible) and refuse to revise their assumptions in the way the book demands. A cold, well-adjusted, pleasant but by no means perfect protagonist is more threatening to the prejudiced reader than a victim.

Thus, in this story, the protagonist's resilience in the face of bereavement, his independence of action, and even daring (his wild midnight behaviour with Kenny), his attacking rather than defensive position in connection with a range of issues (the environment, modern architecture, and university education) all illustrate a strength which means that George cannot be marginalised as 'pathetic' or 'neurotic' or have applied to him any of the other code words by which straights seek to pigeon-hole our varied experiences. He commands respect, not pity. He is not particularly lovable; but he is a force to be reckoned with. For a novel to achieve this – even to attempt it – in 1964 is itself a fact worthy of notice.

Isherwood, however, as I have said, launches a second attack, which is against typical, conformist, heterosexual family life. The novel is not a defence of homosexuality – sexuality is only an issue in so far as it creates paranoia among straights – but an attack on a certain kind of heterosexual lifestyle. (We may be reminded of the way Ivy Compton-Burnett attempts the same task, in much more melodramatic ways, in a score of novels.) This lifestyle is seen as vitiated by an unquestioning acceptance of prevailing ideas and patterns of behaviour, and its outward manifestations are the sterility and ugliness of the architectural and planning disasters, the descriptions of which take up considerable space in the novel. Rigid orthodoxy results in lifelessness; George embodies, by contrast, a spirit of rebellion. In the lives of the Strunks and the Garfeins, underneath the comfort and complacency, there is in fact a fear:

> Oh yes, indeed, Mr Strunk and Mr Garfein are proud of their kingdom. But why, then, are their voices like the voices of boys calling to each other as they explore a dark unknown cave, growing ever louder and louder, bolder and bolder? Do they know that they are afraid?
> No. But they are very afraid.
> What are they afraid of?
> They are afraid of what they know is somewhere in the darkness around them, of what may at any moment emerge into the undeniable light of their flashlamps, nevermore to be ignored, explained away. The fiend that won't fit into their statistics, the gorgon that refuses their plastic surgery, the vampire drinking blood with tactless uncultured slurps, the bad-smelling beast that doesn't use their deodorants, the unspeakable that insists, despite all their shushing, on speaking its name.
> Among many other kinds of monster, George says, they are afraid of little me. (p. 19)

The unspeakable speaking its name is of course an echo of the phrase 'the love that dare not speak its name' and thus places homophobia as central to their fear. But in general, their lives suffer from a condition diagnosed earlier by Erich Fromm, who was writing during the Second World War and under an imperative to explain the allure of fascism for the weak-minded: 'the structure of modern society affects man in two ways simultaneously: he becomes more independent, self-reliant and critical, and he becomes more isolated, alone, and afraid'.[5] These two sets of characteristics go together. Writing, as I now am, from within an Arab society, the lack of the first group of characteristics ensures the lack, also, of the second. It is above all in capitalist 'democracies' where individual isolation and aloneness is most acute, and Isherwood clearly shows that one of its consequences is scapegoating, the sustaining of a mythology of 'the other'.

The vacuity of the whole society is established through the importance it accords to television. The children, especially, are intoxicated by its meretricious glamour and commercialism: 'As soon as they can speak, they start trying to chant the singing commercials' (p. 17). The narrator also points out that young children base their lives on a kind of imitation of what they see on the television. Although this is true, Isherwood has not quite scored the point he thinks he has, for children *always* imitate, and there is little to show that the fatuousness or cultural aridity involved in television or other forms of popular culture is any more damaging or sinister than penny dreadfuls or Victorian sermons. The supposition that contemporary culture is always a decayed or bastardised form of previous purer and better forms is a vulgar superstition of most historical periods.

We have seen that Isherwood does not romanticise George; he is seen as strong, but fallible. In the same way, George's lecture which turns into a disquisition on minorities in society is clearly Isherwood speaking to us directly through his protagonist, but giving us no naïve account of the wholly bad versus the wholly good. Being hated makes people nasty:

> A minority has its own kind of aggression. It absolutely dares the majority to attack it. It hates the majority – not without a cause, I grant you. It even hates the other minorities – because all minorities are in competition; each one proclaims that its sufferings are the worst and its wrongs are the blackest. And the more they all hate, and the more they're all persecuted, the nastier they become! (pp. 54–5)

In putting this view forward, it could be that Isherwood needs to put something negative into the scales, in his fictional assessment of homosexuality, in order to placate anticipated criticism which might consider his depiction of the gay minority too rosy; secondly, it can be viewed as a courageous admission, in so far as it readily provides ammunition for the homophobe who links this 'nastiness' – the effect of being hated – to an innate gay paranoia.

Two components make up the novel's structure: first, it is the story of a single day, described chronologically, so that it begins and ends with George in bed; second, and despite the limitations of the one-day structure, it gives us an account of immensely varied encounters and emotional experiences from George's point of view, in order to bring out the protagonist's complexity of character. (It also provides occasion for authorial statements about prejudice, modernity, family life, and so on.) The novel seems to be offering the tightness of the one-day structure as a kind of propitiation for the otherwise rambling nature of the story, almost as if readers, once they had taken cognizance of this one-day structure, would acquit the novel of any charge of randomness.

The nature of the experiences which the novel sets out to describe are suggested by the ambiguities of the title, *A Single Man*. 'Single' can suggest: bachelor; (newly) bereaved; alone; and, only one man (this last with two contrary senses: powerless because only one; powerful despite being only one). In fact, all these senses are brought out by the rich variety of George's encounters.

His waking, at the beginning of the book, is followed by the morning routine in bathroom and kitchen. It is in this semi-awake state, with his body still barely adjusted anew to movement, that memory lurches to the fore, on George's contemplation of the kitchen doorway, whose narrowness evokes the squeezing past each other of the (then two) dwellers:

> And it is here, nearly every morning, that George, having reached the bottom of the stairs, has this sensation of suddenly finding himself on an abrupt, brutally broken-off, jagged edge – as though the track had disappeared down a landslide. It is here that he stops short and knows, with a sick newness, almost as though it were for the first time: Jim is dead. Is dead. (p. 9)

This stab of memory shows us a vulnerable George. Further memories follow, located in the safe world of childhood:

> Ah, the heartbreakingly insecure snugness of those nursery

> pleasures! Master George enjoying his eggs; Nanny watching him and smiling reassurance that all is safe in their dear tiny doomed world! (p. 11)

This seems to give a promise of a dark and desperate world of adulthood, which the novel seems poised to go on to describe; that this is not really the case, I hope I have sufficiently indicated. George's private communion with himself continues, as he muses over his misuse of books (to send him to sleep, to take his mind off other things), his misanthropy towards children, his encounter with Ruskin sitting on 'the john'.

So varied is the portrait of George that the novel assumes the guise of a systematic investigation of his various traits. The long evening with Charlotte shows him supportive; his sustained, absorbing fantasy of the two semi-naked tennis players, based on the sight of them playing earlier in the day and his lusting after them (their animality contrasting with the artificiality of the car-clogged campus and its phoney rituals); his kindly but futile visit to Jim's ex-flame Doris in the hospital, an old enemy reconciled; his silly mawkish extravaganza with Kenny (this part of the book is especially dated; what George says in his cups might have sounded vaguely sincere in 1964, but we squirm at the Forsterian purple passages now) – all these show a man busy with the business of life, getting on with it, not, in fact, conspicuously in need of radical change, or a replacement for Jim, or indeed anything very particular unless it be the entire transformation of American culture, upon a critique of which this story is fundamentally based.

We can conclude by putting this point in a slightly different way. Although Jim's homosexuality could not be described as merely incidental to the designs of the novel, we can nevertheless imagine a heterosexual figure moving through the same barren landscape without any appreciable difference to the social-protest dimension of the novel. The sexual orientation of George is not obsessively central to the narrator's account, and this results in a matter-of-factness about homosexuality which is positive. It denies that Tennessee Williams scenario of high melodrama (*Cat on a Hot Tin Roof*) where what is purportedly an exposé of bigotry actually keeps the hysterical temperature high and on the boil. Williams takes the high-risk strategy of actually engendering anew revulsion against homosexuality in order to engineer an epiphanic moment of clarity and catharsis, when that revulsion is supposed to be seen to be absurd and delinquent. In the event, bemused and unsubtle audiences of Williams' work often leave the theatre with their revulsion intact. Isherwood, by contrast, assumes as common ground (he knows it *isn't* common ground; it is a ploy, not a conviction) that bigotry is wrong, and by this means hopes to reduce it. (This tactic is very similar to what philosopers of language call 'persuasive definition': for example, one describes one set of combattants in a war as 'terrorists', and the negative attitudes suggested by this term come into being after its deployment, precisely as a result of its deployment.)

A Single Man is not distinguished as a literary work in the way books by Baldwin or Genet, for example, are distinguished. There are no poetic heights, and not much straining beyond the commonplace. Its range is small – so small, that some might be tempted to share Faulkner's attitude of contempt for writings which succeed only because of the pettiness of their ambitions. It is the work of a gentle and perceptive social critic, written in a relatively conventional mode, with good sense and considerable feeling. It deserves attention because, however tame it might now appear, it is one of the very earliest novels to give an emphatically positive face to the gay experience. The tradition of social realism coming out novels, of which Leavitt's *The Lost Language of Cranes,* discussed below, is a superb example, is indebted to the work of Isherwood.

12

Andrew Holleran: *Dancer from the Dance* and *Nights in Aruba*

Andrew Holleran studied history and literature at Harvard University. He then began to study law, but abandoned this in order to be a writer. He attended the University of Iowa Writers' Workshop, did a tour in the Army, and now works and lives in New York City. Dancer from the Dance *(1978) was his first novel, followed by* Nights in Aruba *(1983).*

> *Towards the end, I used to sit on the sofa in the back of the Twelfth Floor [disco] and wonder. Many of them were very attractive, these young men whose cryptic disappearance in New York City their families (unaware they were homosexual) understood less than if they had been killed in a car wreck. They were tall and broad-shouldered, with handsome, open faces and strong white teeth, and they were all dead. They lived only to bathe in the music, and each other's desire, in a strange democracy whose only ticket of admission was physical beauty – and not even that sometimes. All else was strictly classless: The boy passed out on the sofa from an overdose of Tuinols was a Puerto Rican who washed dishes in the employees' cafeteria at CBS, but the doctor bending over him had treated presidents. It was a democracy such as the world – with its rewards and penalties, its competition, its snobbery – never permits, but which flourished in this little room on the twelfth floor of a factory building on West Thirty-third Street, because its central principle was the most anarchic of all: erotic love.*
>
> (*Dancer from the Dance*, pp. 32–3)

Dancer from the Dance (1978)[1] is a re-writing of *The Great Gatsby* by F. Scott Fitzgerald, published in 1925. The story is, superficially at least, entirely different, but if we compare the two novels, both the themes and the style have an enormous similarity. Those familiar with *Gatsby* will, for example, not have failed to hear its echoes in the passage quoted above, especially in the highly lyrical and poetically balanced sentences such as that beginning: 'They lived only to bathe . . .' (We also hear Tennessee Williams.[2])

Both works offer a tone in the narrative which is full of the weary and infinitely sad pursuit by people for a partner, a purpose, an escape from the suffocating sense of meaninglessness. They both portray people in real fear (the sort Fromm speaks of in *The Fear of Freedom*), unable to deal with the multiple choices offered by a modern capitalist 'democracy'. They both combine in a peculiarly satisfying and reassuring way a poignant acceptance of life's inevitable unhappiness with an insistent sense of the need and the possibility of stoical acceptance in the face of that truth. Chekhov comes to mind here, though his prose is much more down-to-earth. Chekhov's battery commander Vershinin in *The Three Sisters* says that people can't be happy, they can only hope to be, and Fitzgerald and Holleran are committed to this view. In the American writers, the pursuit of pleasure, as a way of avoiding or postponing the facing of the truth of life's emptiness, is more pronounced than in Chekhov.[3]

Countless details underline the parallel. Gatsby's famous politeness is duplicated in Holleran's hero, Malone: 'Malone still had only one set of manners, for all people, and they were somewhat too polite for this place' (p. 106). Malone is the subject of fascinating rumours about his past, which add to his attractive mysteriousness, as is Gatsby:

> At first we thought he was a medical student; then we heard he worked on Seventh Avenue for Clovis Ruffin; besides that, he was dying of an incurable bone disease. Then someone said he didn't work at all and was being kept by an Episcopalian bishop; and so Malone went through as many guises as the discotheques we danced at. (p. 111)

As with Coriolanus, all tongues speak of him. (In both novels, the central character is often absent, and in his absence is spoken about with intense curiosity, with which the readers themselves naturally become infected.)

The symbolic importance of clothes in Gatsby (I am thinking of the scene in which Daisy weeps over Gatsby's silk shirts) is also echoed here:

> The clothes! The Ralph Lauren polo shirts, the Halston suits, the Ultrasuede jackets, T-shirts of every hue, bleached fatigues and painter's pants, plaid shirts, transparent plastic belts, denim jackets and bomber jackets, combat fatigues and old corduroys, hooded sweat shirts, baseball caps, and shoes lined up under a forest of shoe trees on the floor; someone had once left the house and all he could tell his friends was that Malone had forty-four shoe trees in his closet. (p. 20)

Malone and Gatsby use conspicuous consumerism as a disguise. Just as the sensationally expensive parties that Gatsby gives at his mansion are noted for the fact that he hardly appears at them himself – they are for show only, to attract back to himself the (in fact unrepeatable) dream of Daisy – so Malone's stylish clothes are not his 'real' clothes at all, but vehicles for making himself a socialite rather than an individual. Fitzgerald's narrator agrees exactly with Holleran's: 'I finally stood up, depressed at all these things [the clothes] – for what were they but emblems of Malone's innocent heart, his inexhaustible desire to be liked?' (p. 21).

It is this boyish innocence which is the strongest similarity between the two characters. Even the sporting metaphors (Fitzgerald was obsessed with football) are similar:

> He always looked like a student who has just come in off the playing fields, eyes glowing from an afternoon of soccer. He always looked like that, even in the depths of a subway station, on the dingiest street in Manhattan. (p. 17)

Innocence eventually results in pain and disillusionment, and Malone's friend Sutherland explains the chief 'flaw' in Malone's character, a flaw shared by Gatsby: '[he is] still searching for love, when it should be perfectly clear to us all by now that there is no Mister Right. . . . We are all alone' (p. 48).

A further similarity is that both characters run their lives on the principle of deferred gratification, at least in the crucial pre-history of each man before the present time of the novels' events. Gatsby spends years and years amassing a fortune and cultivating a style of vulgar flamboyance which he personally dislikes, in the hope that one day Daisy will return to him, attracted like a moth to the light. Malone, in a totally different fashion but with a similar aim, commutes to his deadly job and reads the *New York Times* and is 'responsible' in his community on environment issues, and all the time he is waiting for his life to start. It is not going to start whilst he denies his basic sexual nature and yearns for the heterosexual pattern of life with all its specious stability.

Why should Holleran follow so closely in the footsteps of Fitzgerald? I should say at this stage that, with all the similarities between the two books, there is nothing in the Holleran which would justify one in using the term 'derivative' in its pejorative sense. I have much more the feeling that the later novelist is offering a kind of homage to an earlier master, reworking material in a more modern and specifically gay context. Woody Allen's film *Interiors* is somewhat similar; a film exactly like a film Bergman himself might have made, but actually made by someone else, in the Bergman style, in order to stress that that style is still valid and wonderful and could/should be used by others. (We also need to consider the, to my way of thinking, less likely posibility of a Holleran not actually aware of the parallels with the Fitzgerald, having subsumed the influences of the latter unconsciously.)

All of this leads us to the inevitable view that something about the Gatsby/Malone character must have a fundamental appeal to the United States reader (and presumably others). There are two aspects to this appeal. The first is what I should like to call vacuous plenitude. Despite the massive wealth and corresponding opportunities for leisure and pleasure characterising the United States in this century, personal happiness remains elusive. Abundance is not of itself life-enhancing. Stated baldly this is a truism, but of course what counts in literature is whether truths, however stale, can be rendered real and immediate in the work in question. The flappers of the 1920s in the United States' Jazz Age reappear, in a different guise but with the same hedonistic aim, at the raunchy gay locales of Holleran's New York of the

1970s. And, for them too, life is empty. It is the lost generation all over again.

A second appeal of the two novels is their depiction of innocence in the central characters, who are surrounded by others emphatically the opposite of innocent. The myth of the United States' past is that of breaking away from corrupt old Europe and starting a new clean enterprise on a fresh continent; the notion of innocence is thus central to American culture. Both writers locate innocence – they avoid the preposterous mistake of equating it with sexual experience alone – primarily in the capacity for wonder and hope. Gatsby makes himself ridiculous because he genuinely and immaturely believes that he can re-create the past, carry himself back into it; the novel's final image is of a rower pulling his boat in one direction whilst the river's current, a stronger force, bears him inevitably in the other. Malone's search for true love, or even his belief in it, surrounded as he is by people pursuing one-night stands and having no confidence in anything more enduring, is a version of Gatsby's naivety. For the reader, the possibility of hope in a world manifestly soiled and wretched inevitably lifts the human spirit.

If Malone is the melancholic, his friend Sutherland, vivacious and gregarious, is the epitome of camp humour. I am using 'camp' here to indicate a process of defusing the consequences of the appalling realisation of the world's awfulness. Faced with this, the 'camp' tradition laughs bravely (and/or tastelessly) to anaesthetise the pain. The humour has a defiant assertiveness. For example, here Sutherland replies to a distraught youngster:

> 'You know, I hate being gay,' said the boy, leaning over toward Sutherland, 'I just feel it's ruined my life. It drains me, you know, it's like having a tumor, or a parasite! If I were straight I'd get married and that would be it. But being gay, I waste so much time imagining! I hate the lying to my family, and I know I'll never be any of the things they expect of me,' he said, 'because it's like having cancer but you can't tell them, that's what a secret vice is like.'
>
> Sutherland was speechless at this declaration; he sat there for a moment, with the cigarette holder to his lips, perfectly still; and then he said, 'Perhaps what you *need* . . . perhaps what you need,' he said, in a speculative tone, 'is a good facial.'
>
> (pp. 43–4)

Especially well portrayed in *Dancer* is the gay ghetto; it is a place where we have been pushed, but it is also a place we have chosen for ourselves. A constant theme in contemporary sexual politics' studies is the tragic nature of this missed opportunity. In running away from/being ejected from the nightmare of a banal and trivial heterosexual world, we have systematically and culpably recreated its worst features. Most significantly, human communication is replaced by the enslavement of style and custom and the pursuit of sensation. Holleran's Twelfth Floor Disco has members

> . . . who seemed to have no existence at all outside this room. They were never home, it seemed, but lived only in the ceaseless flow of this tiny society's movements. They seldom looked happy. They passed one another without a word in the elevator, like silent shades in hell, hell-bent on their next look from a handsome stranger. Their next rush from a popper. The next song that turned their bones to jelly and left them all on the dance floor with heads back, eyes nearly closed, in the ecstasy of saints receiving the stigmata. They pursued these things with such devotion that they acquired, after a few seasons, a haggard look, a look of deadly seriousness. Some wiped everything they could off their faces and reduced themselves to blanks. Yet even these, when you entered the hallway where they stood waiting to go in, would turn toward you all at once in that one unpremeditated moment (as when we see ourselves in a mirror we didn't know was there), the same look on all their faces: Take me away from this. Or, Love me. (pp. 30–31)

Holleran returns again and again to this theme of the absence of love. As Sutherland informs Malone, 'There is no love in this city . . . only discotheques' (p. 90). His comment comes in an extended passage the gist of which is that when love has gone there is only dancing and clothes from Bloomingdale's. But as a metaphor, the dance is ambiguous. On the one hand, it epitomises the gay lifestyle at its most meaningless, but on the other hand it carries with it an infectious energy. The need to dance is 'the crazy compulsion with which we resolved all the tangled impulses of our lives . . .' (p. 35). Yet again, we have echoes of Fitzgerald, who at the same time parodies and criticises the vanities of the rich in his fiction whilst (in fiction and his own life) seeing their immense and seductive attraction.

One of the strongest experiences represented in *Dancer* is tiredness; the characters always seem as if they must be exhausted, and there is no let-up in the social whirl. On the other hand, tranquillity is to be found in the 'heterosexual' suburbs (gays always live down town). The suburbs are boring to a degree, but they have enviable certainties, and emotional solidity. Malone feels their attraction poignantly, as if for something irretrievably lost:

> Kids were playing football in the town park, and another football game swept across the high-school field, and boys on bicycles were drawing lazy circles in the supermarket parking lot, and families were out in their backyards raking leaves. It was the sort of scene Malone turned sentimental over. He always passed through Sayville with a lingering regret for its big white houses and friendly front yards with picket fences and climbing roses. He always looked back as he went through, saying this might be that perfect town he was always searching for, where elms and lawns would be combined with the people he loved. But those summer taxis drove inevitably through it, like vans bearing prisoners who are being transferred from one prison to another – from Manhattan to Fire Island – when all we dreamed of, really, in our deepest dreams, was just such a town as this, quiet, green, untroubled by the snobberies and ambition of the larger world; the world we could not quit. (p. 16)

What takes them all past Sayville and into Fire Island is, in the end, sex. This is established from the very beginning of the novel:

> . . . when Stanford [University] sent me a questionaire asking what was the peak experience of the past ten years of my life, a voice inside answered without hesitation: sucking Alfredo Montavaldi's cock. (It certainly meant more than Professor Leon's Chaucer seminar.) (p. 9)

Later, Malone endorses Heine's sentiment that fame is not worth one kiss from a milkmaid. Sutherland tells Malone that in perilous times such as the present 'there are no values to speak of and one can cling to only concrete things – such as cock' (p. 89).

Here is the heart of the matter. Sex might not make one happy – we read of 'faces gloomy with lust' (p. 124) – but at least it is something to cling to.

But beyond sex, even, is time; time as the identified enemy since Shakespeare's sonnet sequence and even earlier. To be sexually attractive is to be winning (not really, of course, but apparently) this battle:

> For what is the real sadness of doomed queens? That they run in packs with one another waiting for the next crow's foot to appear, and wondering how many more seasons they can spend on Fire Island before they have to take a house in up-state New York. (pp. 11–12)

The dancers of the Twelfth Floor are fighting too:

> For what was this room but a place to forget we are dying? . . . Everyone was a god, and no one grew old in a single night. No, it took years for that to happen . . .' (p. 34)

In the exchange of letters introducing the novel, we find the following literary advice:

> I don't think a novel is a historical record; all a piece of literature should do, I think, is tell you what is was like touching Frank Romero's lips for the first time on a hot afternoon in August in the bathroom of Les's Café on the way to Fire Island. (pp. 7–8)

Holleran himself certainly eschews any pretensions in *Dancer* to present a full sociological record of the gay community. Rather, unsystematically and with great skill, he creates through discursive passages and lyrical musings an atmospheric portrait – incomplete and impressionistic, certainly – which is carefully ambiguous. The fun, the parties, the sex and the drugs are all exciting and desired, but they are also indicators of a doomed life (though not necessarily more doomed than the followers of deadly heterosexual routine at Sayville). Like Fitzgerald before him, Holleran sees this kind of life as inevitably involving glamour and squalor together:

> They were bound together by a common love of a certain kind of music, physical beauty, and style – all the things one shouldn't throw away an ounce of energy pursuing, and sometimes throw away a life pursuing. (p. 30)

In Holleran's next novel of gay life, *Nights in Aruba,*[4] Sutherland's Chekhovian stoicism provides the basis for the implied author's view of the world. Thus, Friel, speaking of gays, says that we are 'creatures caught between two kingdoms. That of sea and land. But we mustn't weep, like the little mermaid. We must *make do*' (p. 125). So there is the choice: weep, or make do; no sense of active resistance, or creative engagement with the world. Above all, no sense of personal sufficiency or power to make a difference in the world. This is the major problem with Holleran's whole fictional enterprise. There is a defeatism, a cast of characters who are entirely passive. We wouldn't find *any* of Holleran's characters going on a civil rights' march – they are more likely, especially in this novel, to be sqeezing themselves into a closet and going to Mass to eye up the altar boys, and following social conventions which even the most conventional would surely not allow to loom so large in their daily lives.

They are so completely passive in the face of attack that our credulity is strained. For example, Friel's four brothers won't let him assist in carrying the coffin of his own mother, to whom he was devoted. One of them says to him: 'Because you're a fruit' (p. 212). There is no further comment on this, and one assumes that one is intended to think that Friel accepts this and has no reply. It is difficult to believe, let alone sympathise with, this degree of spinelessness.

The whole book is like something out of the 1950s, apologetic, religious, and blinkered socially, politically, and in fact humanly. *Dancer* is redeemed – indeed, deserves its reputation as among the best gay novels ever written – by its poetic nuances and sensitivities, and the universalising of its themes. *Aruba* is just defeatist. Not in the same vile category as *Boys in the Band,* it nevertheless shares with that play a heterosexist perception of the gay experience: doomed, joyless, compulsive. Here is a typical cruising scene:

> Even on nights when I met someone and went to his apartment

> or brought him to my own, encouraged by success – or simply avaricious – I would return to the park to find someone else. Other nights I found no one, or no one to my liking, and I returned home with my night finally ended by the knowledge that now I could go to bed without that nagging sense of possibilities not taken advantage of. Other nights I stood before my building till someone walked by. The reason I still lived in New York was that someone almost always did, hoping that between himself and his own apartment a lover would spring up out of the pavement and save himself from the dreadful fate of ending his evening alone. (p. 6)

Nevertheless, it has to be admitted that Holleran sees the alternative as equally dire. The inanity of 'ordinary' life is his favourite theme. The narrator's father 'eventually . . . moved to Chicago and went to work for Standard Oil. He gave me two pieces of advice: never to save money on shoes, and to treat oneself to a steak dinner now and then' (p. 31). To the narrator's amazement, Vittorio tells him feebly: 'I want to be successful . . . and have a family' (p. 92). Vittorio settles down to a celibate and closeted and stunted life in Jaspers; meeting the narrator in Jaspers one evening, he says sarcastically: 'Tomorrow we have a big project, however, which will provide a break in the routine. Tomorrow . . . we are going to organise her [his mother's] shoes!' (p. 224).

Vittorio, commenting on the willingness of people to buy encyclopaedias from him because of their boredom and desire to talk to someone, says to Mr Friel, the boss: 'Can you understand the scale, the monumentality of the boredom of most people's lives?' and Friel replies with: 'It only confirms Schopenhauer's dictum that once a man is free of his material needs, he is only confronted with the consciousness of life's essential emptiness' (p. 95).

The unconventional attitudes and behaviour of 'The Clam' certainly place him in the hedonist rather than the boring-and-stable camp. We see this in his misanthropy. He moves from teaching to cleaning the schools because 'I would much rather sweep up after the shits than have to talk to them . . .' (p. 90). Nevertheless, he has a gusto and energy quite unlike the 'doomed queens' of *Dancer*. He approvingly cites the Greeks, who knew what were the best things in life: 'Health, beauty.

Money honestly earned. And . . . To be young with one's friends . . .' (p. 63). His raw hedonism emerges in his talk with Vittorio about 'The Clam's' affair with the army cook. Vittorio is regretting that the cook doesn't admire 'The Clam' for his mind and his personality. 'The Clam' replies that the best part of *no one* is their mind, and rapsodises about the cook's body: ' . . . that snow-white stomach, that gorgeous ass, that pendulous dick!' (p. 87).

The contrast between the worlds of excitement and stable routine are sometimes humorously contrasted:

> Wheatworth answered the telephone one evening in his apartment, picking it up with his free hand while the other remained in the rectum of the bartender who lay on the bed beside him, head back, gasping, and heard his mother say, 'Hi! Your father just said I should give you a ring. He's sitting across from me now. He watches TV from the small sofa instead of the big one now.' (p. 103)

Love, and the search for it, seem to be the only way out of life's *impasse.* But even here there is a problem; without love there is loneliness, but with love there is a fear of declining into banality: 'It was as if I longed to be rescued from my banal life by Love, and then, once having obtained the object, found a new form of banality stretching before us: that of lovers' (p. 108). Once again, there is a close Chekhovian parallel; the doctor in *The Three Sisters* says something very similar.

The bad news of this novel is not confined to the small social groupings discussed, but widens out to embrace the whole human delinquency. 'The world', in its journalistic sense, is a terrible place, and we are reminded of this fact through the media each day, and thus each day in our daily lives we have reinforced within our minds a general sense of human aimlessness and depravity:

> I bought the next day's *Times* at the drugstore the moment the truck delivered it, and went up to my room. I read a while: the article on the Chinese census, unemployment in Puerto Rico, a man who wrapped furniture in linen, an exposé of white chocolate, and the tiny paragraphs that told – on an obscure page – of murders, stabbings, bodies found in Central Park, the

baby thrown out a window in Brooklyn by a mother convinced he was the devil. Then I set the alarm and lay down and composed myself to sleep. But sleep was impossible. (p. 7)

Aruba has many of the fine, one might say marvellous, features of *Dancer*; it uncannily portrays, not merely in individual passages but as it were indirectly through an accumulation of mood, style, modes of speech and register, a sense of desolate loneliness. Some of the techniques for doing this are actually rather simple: the narrator's name is never given; his friends (most of them, those other than the novel's main characters) are referred to in passing even when the narrator is with them, strongly suggesting that he is not *really* with them. They thus appear soulless adjuncts of his life.

The idyll with Sal is over because the narrator refuses to *say* that he is Sal's 'lover' (Sal wants monogamy, and gets it with someone else quite soon in Fort Worth) and pushes him into the arms, or at least the friendships of, other men, because he doesn't want Sal to be too dependent. Then he spends years thinking of what he is missing without having him. All this dithering and uncertainty provides another example of the inability of the narrator (and therefore, impliedly, Everygayman) to achieve serenity or peace unless they are stupid. On this last point, much is made of the fact that Sal never reads because 'It makes me fall asleep' (p. 200) and this is meant to be a terrific joke at Sal's expense. But it is also a comment on the narrator's supposed status as 'educated', which is never on show but always to be taken for granted, and which prevents contentment. Actually, as I am trying to argue, whatever cultural impedimenta he carries round in his head, he is morally and emotionally primitive – stupid, if you will – and the laugh is on him. The Sal/ignorant syndrome also links in with the whole Western literary tradition of culture = emasculation, unculture = virility.

Despite the many parallels with *Dancer*, the later novel is very much inferior. What in the first book was a fresh exciting novel, here becomes routine, jaundiced, repetitive. The tired quality comes out in the prose, which lacks the gorgeous inventiveness, inspired sparkle and mythic dimension of Dancer. There is also a strange toleration of Christianity. This may be a difference between United States and British readers. I certainly find it extraordinary to find that Christianity in general, and Catholicism in particular, are represented as only mildly exceptionable. The view seems to be that if it shrugged off its old-fashioned attitudes to sexuality, and perhaps made some radical adjustments to its theology, it would be all that could be wished. To describe in this way what, for gays worldwide, is one of the most repressive systems of belief is rather shocking.

Examples of this attitude can be seen in the warmth with which 'Father Bob' is portrayed, and the fact that the central gay characters – especially Friel, Vittorio and the narrator – all go to church (though not, conspicuously, to Communion). Again, Friel sees the Roman Catholic attitude to his sexuality as very little more than something preventing him from making a sincere confession: ' . . . the Church considers *it* a sin, and I don't' (p. 140). The tone is matter-of-fact.

Aruba is also noticeably more sentimental and/or clichéd than *Dancer*:

> We might be joined beyond the grave, and we might not. There might or might not be some moment of forgiveness for everything. (p. 239)

> All that winter I seemed to be an actor taking a part that had been given him for no reason he could discern: I was happy. I kept searching for explanations but in the end there weren't any. (p. 200)

> I ran past the bakery managed by a married couple just shutting up the cash register, blessing them in my heart because Sal and I bought doughnuts there . . . (p. 198)

Friel asks the narrator what is his 'cross' because, as he says, every Catholic must have one (itself a cliché):

> 'Why?' I said. 'Why must there be a cross?'
> 'Why must there be a penis?' he said, turning at the top of the stairs. (p. 126)

In fine, *Aruba*, compared to *Dancer*, is less interesting and more obsessional about age, death and approaching death, grey hair, the envying of youth, the slow decline of erotomania with the onset of middle age; and seeing life as *simply* a process of dying, a view so indulgent and repellantly negative that one yearns for a D. H. Lawrence figure to come round the corner with some exhilarating affirmation of life. Here is a typical passage:

> Shortly after parting [from friends] you realised you had done nothing but extract a dull set of facts. What you really wanted to know was if there was any progress, any evolution, any goal toward which you were all moving. In fact you were simply growing older. (p. 116)

If we take an obvious, and rather literal-minded approach, we can say that Holleran's world offers a choice between juicy sex, drugs and parties, or a serene evening with the fatuous world of TV soap operas. This stark choice is repeatedly emphasised. Neither of the books contains hints of any of those things providing life-enhancing joy to all those for whom the above two activities do not represent the entire catalogue of possibilities: friendship, love, the intellectual life. The attitude is summed up thus: ' . . . the nights I used to spend dancing or walking the streets, I now spent in bed reading *The New York Times*' (p. 235).

The novel also wallows in reactionary political and social attitudes, as well as a thrusting to the fore of values based on self-pity, passivity, resignation, conventionality, inaction, and pessimism. It is as if the famous Byron/Shelley debate, ranging dark cynicism against affirmative optimistic quasi-Utopianism – a question not quite settled in *Dancer* – has here been definitively settled in favour of Byron. In the narrator himself there is a pathetic lack of resolve to act, to make his own life:

> I wanted to be free of the family and their judgment and expectations. The summons to a reunion was like the summons to a funeral. I wanted to stay in the city instead and eschew the obligatory and tedious customs. (p. 237)

But of course he allows these customs to hold sway. On another occasion, he lies to his mother and pretends to her that he goes to church regularly whilst in New York. He is shocked that a woman he meets doesn't want a baby unless the father undertakes to bring it up:

> The chill that spread through me on hearing these words made

> me realise that, while homosexual, I was a completely conventional person at the same time, like the man who, after a night of sexual debauch, joins his family at Thanksgiving and is horrified to learn that his niece is chewing her nails. (p. 160)

The narrator's closetry is typical. He doesn't even tell his parents about being gay, even when middle aged. When asked outright by his mother if he's homosexual, we get: 'I jumped up from the sofa, said, "No! Of course not!" in a voice as sharp as my father's when he was angry, and left the room' (p. 156). This in the early 1980s.

Even the narrator's love for his parents puts us off because it is described in a clichéd manner; it is unconvincing, in that even Catholics don't reproach themselves this much; and it manages to be sentimental. It is also condescending:

> I was filled with a sense of disloyal selfishness as I flew north. I turned to the window and said to its scratched glass, 'My parents are dying. They've done nothing wrong, they've been generous and good and loving, and they're sitting in a house in Florida turning old.' (p. 66)

The implied attitude towards the elderly here is that their lives are nothing except the wait for death. This condescension is not confined to the old. Elsewhere he says of a gay couple in New York that they seemed 'as sad as middle-aged women who no longer dress smartly and who go out to their clothesline in their robes during the day' (p. 178). There is no sense that the implied author believes in the possibility that for some women this is a beneficial and liberating change, that the abandonment of the need to 'keep up' and be fashionable is a milestone in the maturity of the individual.

In different degrees, and with different levels of artistic success – there is a wide gap in my view, as I have suggested above, between the very fine first novel and the poor later one – Holleran offers us a dark view of the world; one in which we are as children lost in a wood. Occasionally, in *Aruba,* Holleran recaptures that wonderful ability to encapsulate in an image a felt truth, and then express it elegantly:

> I realised that so much memory and desire swirl about in the

hearts of men on this planet that, just as we can look at Neptune and say it is covered with liquid nitrogen, or Venus and see a mantle of hydrochloric acid, so it seemed to me that were one to look at Earth from afar one would say it is covered completely with Ignorance. (p. 240)

13

David Leavitt: *The Lost Language of Cranes*

David Leavitt (1961–) was raised in California and graduated from Yale University. He now lives in East Hampton, New York. His fiction has appeared in the New Yorker, Harper's *and* Christopher Street. *His first book was a collection of short stories entitled* Family Dancing. The Lost Language of Cranes *is his first novel.*

The Lost Language of Cranes[1] is an outstanding example of the recent tradition of coming out novels, many examples of which appeared in the 1970s and 1980s. The formula normally used in such novels involves, first, showing us the family relationships before the coming out, then the more or less traumatic coming out period itself, and finally, some time later, we see whether and to what extent the family/friends have adapted to the new information. *The Lost Language of Cranes* conforms to this pattern, but in a particularly fine and perceptive way which makes it exemplary of the genre.

The difficulties for a gay novelist portraying these confrontations start not with problems of aesthetic choice but personal pain; for however dissimilar are the specific characters and circumstances in the fictional story, and whatever distancing techniques are employed by the author in avoiding the autobiographical and in the inventing of entirely different scenarios, the core of the scene, if well done, will depict and explore feelings which, one can say with confidence, he has experienced himself. In the lives of gay men, there is of course a wide spectrum of experience, running from, let us say, a parental reaction of disgust, rejection, ejection from the home, and physical violence, to the nervously half-concealed anxiety of the ultra-liberal father and mother who will 'accept' their son with a facial pallor and tremulous voice giving the lie to their words. At the worst, there is emotional and physical banishment and a threat of bodily harm; at the very best, the most fortunate of us have been 'policed by embarrassment'.[2] Put another way, in so far as, given a choice, they would always opt for their children to be straight, parents are *per se* the enemy. It is, of course, not accidental that the most virulent anti-gay campaigns put themselves forward not in this negative way but as pro-family. Indeed, being pro-family has become a euphemism for, *inter alia,* homophobia.

Then, to hold the pen steady and, through the act of writing, force oneself to revisit the sites of a pain which, if now numbed and incorporated into the person (like a body's habituating itself to some chronic but minor dysfunction) vigorously renews itself in that act of writing, is a courageous and difficult task. The writing is a second coming out; certainly the conditions are more favourable, but dangers remain.

These are as follows. First, a kind of furiously indignant separatism: all heterosexuals are our enemies, their institutions, practices and conduct rebarbative. We must have no truck with them. This is an easy, understandable, and for some, irresistible choice. (The way in which, in matters of racism, Baldwin manages to avoid it whilst at the same time piling high before our eyes all the facts which, one would think, would be sure to lead him to adopt it, is a major component in his writing, one most plainly seen in *The Fire Next Time.*[3] The opposite cases are Malcolm X, Eldridge Cleaver and George Jackson, dripping with venom.) To adopt Wordsworth's dictum 'that we have all of us one human heart',[4] to follow Godwin in his denunciation of sectaries and his insistence on universal benevolence, is hard.

plitting up into rival gangs, organising struggles against clear and declared opponents, is easier; and it is how the world goes. The gay novel which eschews this partisanship gives us a wider view. It does not lessen our anger or compromise our determination, but it helps us to avoid the us/them polarity on which the very bigots we wish to attack, thrive.

The second danger is to offer a kind of implied apology for gayness; some recent novels fall into this trap, issuing from sensibilities so well trained that they adopt the establishment viewpoint and feel a need to justify their own.

Leavitt's novel offers a finely observed coming out scene

avoiding both these dangers. It starts with the gay son, Philip, in his twenties, visiting the parental home at a time when his mother, Rose, is engrossed in a television book serialisation. Steeling himself to declare his sexuality, Rose's first words, as he asks for her attention, reflect her irritation at being interrupted in her viewing: 'Be quiet, something important's happening' (p. 168). Indeed it is – or is about to – but in the real world she would rather not think about, plunged as she is in her escapist television drama. Apart from this opening irony, we notice that a truly pivotal moment is juxtaposed with the mundane. This sense of sameness – it is a day like any other – makes it harder for Philip to generate the will to say something importantly different. After all, he has had countless opportunities in the past to say what he has to say, but the breaking through of that settled daily humdrum, which he hopes his words will demolish, comes hard.

Philip's opening line is, 'I have something to say to you' (p. 168). This is corny, but at moments of emotional intensity, linguistic felicity and carefully chosen *mots justes* do not come easily. Then there is a rigmarole about whether he would like to sit down or to stand – something which is never inquired into when familial relaxedness is present. Then 'Here goes' (another nervous, making-it-worse ominous phrase) and finally 'I'm gay' *with his eyes closed.* This last is also a fine touch; for whatever these liberal parents might find it in themselves to say to live up to his highest expectations, he wants to avoid seeing what he is sure is going to be a wincing shock. If you do not see, you can pretend afterwards that perhaps it never took place.

Rose, we now discover, had once found gay porn under Philip's bed but, with the customary human skill in excluding evidence which does not fit neatly into a prefabricated view of the world to which, each with a different view, all of us cling tenaciously, she ascribes its presence to a joke present from a friend, or something her son must have found in the garbage.

Leavitt goes on to give us a convincing account of the mild and plausible homophobia found in such parents. To Philip's plea, following the received wisdom of the post-Spock era, that 'it's better to be honest', Rose asks: 'Better for whom?' (p. 171). Her view is that there are some areas of the human heart best left unexposed:

I don't believe that just because something's by definition a

> secret it therefore by definition has to be revealed. Keeping certain secrets secret is important to – the general balance of life, the common utility. (p. 173)

When Philip points out that *she* would be quite unable to live in a society in which her heterosexual love were a secret, she resorts to that tired riposte used by those who have exhausted their argumentative ammunition: 'It's not the same' (p. 173). (The whole novel is saying, repeatedly, successfully and with quiet power that it *is* the same.)

Rose's view is somewhat linked to another that she advances: that Philip's gayness is part of contemporary youth's desire for gratification, instead of a commitment to duty. The link between these two arguments is that both are based on the idea of gayness as some kind of indulgence, a sort of pleasure additional to those routinely allotted in this world to the fortunate. Philip's reply is: 'being gay isn't just – gratifying some urge. It's a matter of your life' (p. 173) and he adds, 'My sexuality, my attraction to men, is the most crucial, most elemental force in my life, and to deny it, to pretend it wasn't there because I was afraid of what people would think – that would be a tragedy' (p. 174).

When painful discussions of this kind take place between parents and their children, it is always known and felt that a physical gesture, a hug, is the way to heal and console. Rose, too, knows this, 'but the best she could manage was a bitter little laugh' (p. 171). There is an ambiguity in 'manage' – how far is she being wilful, how far simply incapable for the moment of embracing Philip? – but in general Leavitt is indulgent with Rose, asking us to see her as much a victim of conventions as a stalwart follower of them.

Nevertheless, the failure to hug is, for all its apparent slightness, a betrayal; and this links in neatly with the major irony of the episode. Owen himself is gay, has married Rose and lived a closeted existence, surreptitiously visiting porn cinemas on Sundays, and wholly failing to establish a truly satisfying relationship with his wife. According to Rose's logic, Philip should reject the life of 'gratification' and settle down to heterosexual marriage; in the process making both himself and his wife as sexually unfulfilled and quietly unhappy as Rose herself and Owen. Rose wants to insist on precisely those conventions of which she is, unwittingly, a major casualty.

But her discovery of Owen's sexuality follows speedily. In the scene with Philip, Owen is silent; for he too is a betrayer. He tells his son that Philip's being gay is 'okay' (p. 175) which statement implies he is speaking as a heterosexual. Owen begins to weep; soon it is uncontrollable, and he takes refuge in the shower, so that the noise of the water will mask his sobs. The shower is, of course, a closet. It has been established as such because it is the place in which, lying on the floor and behind closed doors, Philip masturbated as an adolescent. Like his father, he too left the water running to cover the noise. It is at this point, as Rose tries the knob of the door and finds it locked, that 'the truth hit her with all the irrevocable force of a revelation' (p. 177)

Setting up his readers for a scene of son coming out to parents, Leavitt provides a marvellously appropriate second, forced, disclosure about the father. This is linked to a kind of nemesis for Rose: she thinks Philip should stay in his closet, and now she finds her husband has himself lived there all the time, blighting her life as a result.

Philip's coming out experiences are paralleled in those of Jerene, Eliot's black lesbian room-mate. In both cases, what might appear at first glance to be a plethora of unnecessary background details, provided for us by Leavitt, becomes a skilful exercise in 'placing' the lesbian/gay theme within an overall and wholly convincing picture, which includes racism, peer pressure, habit, personal hypocrisies and the desire to conform. We truly learn about these people before we see their homophobic prejudice, and this helps us understand.

Jerene's parents by adoption are rich; the father is a succesful lawyer. Their desire is to integrate into White society, and to become 'accepted', which of course involves accepting the moral values which underpin that society – values which are responsible amongst other things for the racism from which they both suffer. Their situation is the same as that of lesbians/gays who accept the trammelling of their culture, their sense of personal identity, their very hearts' desires – they accept the public desecration of this in return for a place in the sun: as a judge, a Christian minister, even a small-time businessman, or a 'respectable' wife and mother. (We are reminded here of the Baldwin of *Another Country*, investigating the complex relationship between homophobia and racism, and Black people's acceptance or otherwise of gay people, and what precisely this means.) It is the old story of bad faith, and Leavitt is concerned to show how expensive it is. For example, in an early scene the parents visit an elegant restaurant where even the black waitresses 'gave the family curious, condescending glances, as if to question whether they belonged there'. But they stick it out, 'pretending enjoyment as if their lives depended on it, and in certain ways their lives did depend on it' (p. 57).[5]

Jerene's parents make explicit the sentiment that, in the case of Jean Genet, is agonisingly potent even when left unvoiced: the reminder to the child that s/he is a recipient of charity, than which little can be more frightening, for it is in the nature of conferred favours that they can be withdrawn at any time: 'You would've grown up mighty differently if we hadn't come along' (p. 58) her mother tells her; and her father says, 'Just be glad you've got all this . . .' (p. 60), but the girl is not fooled. She knows that 'None of it was hers except by refugee's luck' (p. 60).

The father's capitulation to mainstream United States' values is best illustrated in his becoming a Nixon delegate at the Republican party convention in 1968; for a few seconds of glory, he is in front of the TV cameras explaining why a Black man should vote for a Republican. (He is granted temporary celebrity only because he has 'abandoned' his race.) The mother is not, unsurprisingly, impressed by her husband's words to camera ('I fully believe that Richard Nixon is what our country and our economy needs now' – p. 61) but deeply excited by the fact of his being on television. She tells Jerene: 'Hush up. . . . How many times in your life are you gonna get to see your father on television?' (p. 61). In all the predictable details of daily life, father and mother attempt to smother Jerene's individuality. Jerene's playing basketball, for example, or refusing to wear pretty dresses, are construed as unfeminine and therefore dangerously rebellious. Both are, of course, hostile to separatism, believing in working through the existing system. The father's bland explanation of his position, 'We're all human' (p. 63), is brilliantly characterised as 'wrapping his snobbery and defeat in the guise of Christian good will . . .' (p. 63).

With this background, the emotional deformity revealed by these parents in the coming out scene follows naturally, without any sense of the exaggerated or histrionic. The father's 'I would rather you had told me you were dying of terminal cancer' is matched by the mother's 'It's like a death. . . . As if she's died'

(p. 64) and it is hardly surprising that, after this decisive rupture, when Jerene is finally persuaded to phone her mother to try to begin to heal the rift, the latter is able to say, 'I don't know anyone named Jerene . . . You must have the wrong number' (p. 65). On one level, this is just a cruel response; but on another it represents a literal truth. For the mother, sexual conformity is so basic that it is tied up inextricably with identity; a daughter who has revealed 'this filth, this abomination' (p. 64) starts the process by which both parents are able, indeed have an urgent psychological need, to reject and deny their belonging to Jerene. Their implied threat – that an adopted child can always be abandoned, left to its own devices – has come about.

Comparing the two sets of parents, we can see that Leavitt is keen to present us with portraits of both the hysterically and the subduedly hostile, and to give full explanations in the background social milieux of the two sets to explain their differences and their similarities. We notice once again – something strongly borne out in actual life – the extraordinary resilience and tolerance of the rejected children. It is an important observation that those whom society has chosen to oppress with a weight of guilt will, at some level, feel that guilt, however busy their intellects will be in dismissing the spurious reasons which are offered to justify that guilt. It may be the case that this guilt renders such children reluctant to judge their parents harshly, to extend to them, rather, a gentle solicitude. Thus, Philip has no fear of being rejected, but 'He was afraid only of the power he held to hurt her' (p. 110)

The coming out dramas of the novel are central; but they are only dramatic expressions of a general social and familial malaise which has its roots in sexual dishonesty. Rose and Owen spend half a lifetime together without admitting to each other that they have each been unfaithful. When Rose bumps into Owen on his Sunday wanderings (the day he steals off to the porn cinema), her experience of seeing him in an unwonted context makes him seem a complete stranger, and underlines the fact that there are areas of feeling and experience which they are unable to share with each other: 'She thought, Twenty-seven years of marriage, and I hardly know him' (p. 19).

Owen keeps an emotional distance from his son, depriving him of paternal warmth and support, because he is afraid that 'if he got too close to his son, things might rub off on Philip – things he preferred not to name.' Thus Leavitt delineates the moral cowardice behind so many of these problems, leading to separation:

> sitting across from each other at breakfast . . . it was as if the white kitchen table were an Arctic tundra stretching between them, vast and insurmountable. There was no tension, no suppressed anxiety; there was just miles and miles of nothing. (p. 128)

Ex-Catholics frequently tell you how, whilst passing some government office or imposing building, they will unthinkingly genuflect in front of its doors, so ingrained has habit become. In the same way, Leavitt shows the intensity of adolescent sexual guilt as experienced by gays; for Philip as an adult can be forced back into the era of repressed youth if the props are right, as shown in this moment when his mother enters his bedroom unannounced:

> He flew into the air so fast that the book he was reading leapt out of his hand, hitting a wall. Only after a few seconds did he realize that the worst nightmare of his adolescence was not coming true; that he had been caught in the act of nothing for which Rose might find him guilty; that he was sitting surrounded not by pornographic magazines, but by the books of his childhood, the most innocent books of all. (p. 116)

Leavitt's anatomy of sexual dishonesty often carries additional conviction when a wry humour is employed; for the humour defuses rather than inflames our moral outrage, making us uneasily acquiesce in the recognition of human delinquency without quite bringing us to disgust. Thus, Jerene's grandmother, Nellie, whose family wants to 'protect' her from the news that Jerene is a lesbian, is told that her granddaughter went to Africa and had a family!

The chief difference which emerges between Philip and Owen is that of honesty versus dishonesty, openness and closetry. When Owen, making his early tentative steps into the world of truth, tells his son that everyone is basically bisexual, Philip recognises more shuffling. This stance, he says, 'can become an excuse, a way of avoiding committing yourself, or admitting the truth. It means you can duck out when the going gets rough' (p. 232)

Despite this father/son contrast, Philip is by no means perfect. His relationship with Eliot breaks up – the latter abandons him – because Philip is constantly clinging, needing reassurance. With the experience of many of those who have been traumatised as children, he cannot bring himself to believe that he will ever be loved, or found lovable.

Reversing the mainstream literary tradition, whereby heterosexual families represent the healthy norm from which homosexual partnerships are seen as a drastic falling off, Leavitt offers us the gay 'marriage' of Derek Moulthorp and Geoffrey Bacon as, if not an ideal, then at least one in which a child, Eliot, has been reared surrounded by love and uncontaminated by that noxious atmostphere that gay youth is forced to inhale in every 'normal' home. Heterosexual readers will certainly see this as a literary equivalent of 'gesture politics' – an artificial device to oversimplify, and make what might appear to be a facile point. In fact, *any* positive images of gay relationships will always appear forced to such readers, because they start from the initial and erroneous premise (consciously or not) that such relationships usually fail.

Actually, Leavitt contrasts this positive, stable and loving gay couple with those aspects of gay culture which have beeen found heartless and arid by gay and straight alike. The scenes of anonymous sex in booths and cinemas are done with great skill and directness. Here is Owen in the cinema:

> The man wanted to go somewhere else. He sat hunched in his chair, his fly open, an erection tenting his underwear. He looked at Owen. 'I have a place nearby; we could go there,' he said, and Owen opened his mouth and looked the other way. He imagined saying yes, imagined how they would have to walk out of the theatre, exchange names, perhaps shake hands; how they would have to talk about their jobs and lives on the way to wherever they were going (what could he say?); worst of all, how they would have to admit to each other in the broad light of day that they had come, each alone, to that dark room on Third Avenue, that heart of shame and lonely self-indulgence, and thereby acknowledge each other as human beings and not just shadows that float in a theatre and mimic, moment by

> moment, the flickering gestures of giants on a screen. Owen knew how to touch; with his hands he could be gentle, fierce, seductive. But in fifteen years of coming to this theatre he had never uttered a word to one of his partners; he hardly knew where to begin. (p. 24)

There are two further scenes in which Philip allows men in the dark to grope in his trousers, whilst in his eyes there are tears of utter loneliness; and one, combining poignancy and comedy, in which Owen phones the 'Macho Man' organisation for an erotic telephone conversation. There is an amusing contrast between the preamble – polite talk about which credit cards are accepted – and the conversation proper, which has the automaton impersonal raunchiness of hired sex. It is amusing, too, to us as readers, because we are embarrassed but nevertheless willing voyeurs of words which can only retain their sexual force within the fantasy context; outside that, they are merely risible:

> After a few minutes the phone rang.
> 'Yeah, this is Bruce.'
> Owen laughed involuntarily. 'Hi, Bruce.'
> 'What's your name, cocksucker?'
> 'Bowen'
> 'Asslicker. You want to suck my cock?' Bruce said.
> Owen took another gulp of bourbon. 'Sure,' he said.
> 'You better do better than "Sure,"' Bruce said. "Cause I want it bad.' He growled. 'I'm sitting here in my hardhat, I just got off an asskicking day at the site. I've got on my oldest pair of jeans, my cock is aching, it's so hard inside my jock. My wife won't go near me. I ain't had a piece of ass for weeks. You know how that makes your cock feel?' (p. 221)

Leavitt astutely picks up the key elements of gay pornography here. The emphasis is on manual labour and rough trade. Middle-class professions, as also culture and learning, suggest a diminution of virility. (Joe Orton, when out cruising, never revealed to his pick-ups that he was a writer; he used to tell them he was a lorry driver.) There is the gay man's (inevitably hopeless, and therefore all the more charged) desire for the straight man, who, notwithstanding, might turn to men in certain circumstances, usually associated with women's supposed unadventurousness in sexual acts, or their unavailability ('My wife won't go near me'). This desire is of course a kind of self-contempt because, by definition, it places gay men themselves outside the group of the desirable. In the same conversation, a minute later, Bruce tells Owen: 'oh yeah, that feels good, you fairy cocksucker' (p. 222); the fantasy is that the gay man submits to the 'real' (= straight) man, experiences his contempt ('fairy') which pleasingly and masochistically reflects his self-contempt, but at the same time is enjoying sexual congress with the straight man. Owen's initial nervous laugh – this is Philip's response, too, in the cinema – soon turns to tears. The impersonality of it is too much for him; it is a point in his favour.

Leavitt feels that he must be comprehensive – that is, the sordid must be balanced by the fine, just as the casual relationships must be offset with depictions of stability – because the novel will be judged as a rounded portrait of gay life, and the fewer there are of these portraits, the more representative and accurate each of them is expected to be. It is a common dilemma experienced in all minority cultures when individuals within that culture begin the task of reclaiming their own truths and speaking with their own authentic voices.

Thus, the sordidness is contrasted with scenes of lyrical sensitiveness. Leavitt evokes Owen's frustrated desire:

> the longing to touch and be touched by another man [began] again its plaintive wail inside him. . . . It was no longer a matter of choice. (p. 132)

The fleeting moment of his meeting with the man in the porn cinema leads to a touchingly adolescent infatuation:

> He was in love with Alex Melchior, with all he knew of him, his underwear and his voice and his telephone number. . . . Hope had stolen into his life just as he was growing comfortable with despair. (p. 133)

The wry humour here gives the description poignancy, whilst preventing the writing from sliding into mawkishness. Early in the novel, Philip abandons a sexual session with Eliot in order to do the dishes. Thus, the novel is prepared to associate sex with cosiness and domesticity, as well as with the sinister raunchiness of impersonal sex. Brad's desire 'to find someone he could settle down with, live with forever' (p. 194) is another antidote to the popular image of gay sexuality.

To emphasise that gay sexuality has this warmth, the novel portrays sex with a sense of humour – something exactly opposite to the spirit of 'pornographic' sex (there is no laughter in blue movies):

> The night wore on towards dawn. Rob was enormously excited, much more excited than Philip himself. Philip thought this to be impolite on his part . . . 'A football player lives next door,' Rob whispered just before Philip came. 'Try to be quiet.' (p. 203)

The humour signals a little corner of triumphant affirmation, for the football player represents the dark side against which the lovers' lives will always be pitched: the intolerant 'macho' male who poses the constant threat of disdain and physical violence.

The novel's important preoccupation with different forms of love and sexual relationships is set in a culture whose details are only sparsely coloured in, but whose general vacuity is suggested by the recurring motif of television. Philip's mother is seen to be so glued to the television screen that she cannot attend to what her son has to tell her, however important it might be. The more extreme case of Jerene's grandmother Nellie – a kind of Rose in a more advanced state of soap opera addiction – reveals how television culture supplants concern for one's own family in favour of the safe, fictional ones on the screen. As Tennessee Williams pointed out in connection with cinema, all the people sit in the dark, passively, and allow a handful of players to act out a vicarious set of experiences for all the people in America. Nellie can hardly bear to wait between episodes, so painfully keen is her experience of the suspense concerning what is going to happen next. Nellie recounts how another of the inmates of the home wrote to the broadcasting network for advance information about whether things eventually turned out okay for two fictional characters, 'in case she died before she found out' (p. 266). In her own case, 'The weekend that Jenny was on the operating table I couldn't sleep a wink' (p. 267). The phrasing suggests that Nellie's life is in limbo between episodes, giving her the sense that the hour or so of fictional time which spans two episodes, during which the operation takes place, is transformed for her into a hugely protracted alternative fiction, in which Jenny is assumed to be lying on the operating table between the Friday night and the show's next installment on Monday.

It is not only the vulgarity and triviality of the soap opera, or its use by 'addicts' to evade the genuinely anguished and responsible choices required of real families, which Leavitt wishes to underline. He also makes the point that conferring this kind of importance on a popular cultural artefact is part of the insidious process by which people relinquish individually exercised discretion. We bow to the implied moral and other codes of televised families rather than thinking for ourselves.

The novel's title stems from two sources. The first is the story unearthed in Jerene's researches, concerning young twins who had developed between themselves a private language: the social workers had decided to split up the twins in order to facilitate their entry into the common linguistic community, but it was an anguished choice because it involved the breaking of a precious and intimate relationship. (Rather the same dilemma faces the psychiatrist Dysart in Peter Shaffer's play *Equus*, for in 'treating' the boy who has blinded six horses, he risks stifling all that is individual, unique, rebellious, visionary, at the same time as he returns the patient to functional normality.)

The second source of the title is based on another 'case study' discovered by Jerene: an abandoned baby alone in a deserted building comes to believe that the mechanical crane outside the window is its mother, and makes screeching noises and staccato movements in pathetic imitation of its supposed parent. Jerene reads this story as exemplifying the need for variety and individuality to be acknowledged in love:

> For each, in his own way, she believed, finds what it is he must love, and loves it; the window becomes a mirror; whatever it is that we love, that is who we are. (p. 183)

Both the private language and the crane-mother stories represent the presence of individual uniqueness, and people's need to express themselves however weirdly that expression might seem to others. Like Laura's glass menagerie, the unusual loves tend to be fragile and are sometimes broken by strangers, especially well-meaning ones. (Jim, in *The Glass Menagerie*, speaks a little in the tone of the social workers whom we can imagine separating the twins in the story for their own good.) To a large extent, of course, we are bound to infer that the oddity of the twins and the crane-child stand as metaphors for gay people, whose oddity – on this reading of the novel's symbolism – should be tolerated. Although the two images are powerful, this is rather unfortunate for it portrays homosexuality as freakish.

The novel's ending is equivocal. Owen has left his wife, but is it a temporary flight, or a determination to live more honestly and openly as a gay man? It is also uncertain whether Philip has found a long-term mate in Brad, although Leavitt uses a stock literary device in order to suggest that the answer is yes: Brad is the man with whom he has been friends for some time – each of them has been separately pursuing some ideal love – without at all considering him as a possible sexual partner. The discovery of this possibility then becomes all the sweeter. (The *locus classicus* of this situation is the relationship between Emma and Mr Knightley in Austen's *Emma*.) The uncertainties about the future of the characters' lives gives the novel a kind of further authenticity for, in the world outside fiction, we do not arrive at conclusive moments; rather, we are always on the brink of a new departure and a new uncertainty. And love's energies are restless: 'the heartstrings yearn to be plucked at any cost, the soul tires of contentment, the body craves any kind of change, even decimation, even death' (p. 47).

Notes

Notes to Chapter 1

1. Ian Ousby (ed.), *The Cambridge Guide to Literature in English* (Cambridge: Cambridge University Press, 1988) p. 114.
2. David Rees, *The Milkman's On His Way* (London: Gay Men's Press, 1982).
3. John Osborne, review in *Bête Noir*, no. 1 (Autumn 1984) p. 101.
4. See, for example, *Literary Theory: An Introduction* (Oxford: Blackwell, 1983).
5. *London Review of Books*, 26 November 1987.
6. Quoted in *Atlantis*, no. 26, June 1988, p. 23.
7. *London Review of Books*, 10 December 1987, p. 19.
8. Andrew Field, *Nabokov. His Life in Part* (London: Hamish Hamilton, 1977) p. 48.
9. Paul Zweig, *The Making of the Poet* (Harmondsworth: Penguin, 1987).
10. Ibid., p. 190.
11. Ibid., p. 188.
12. Quoted in Gregory Woods, *Articulate Flesh* (New Haven, Conn.: Yale University Press, 1987) p. 138.
13. Tom Marshall, *The Psychic Mariner: A Reading of the Poems of D. H. Lawrence* (London: Heinemann, 1970) p. 128.
14. John Logan, *Hart Crane: 'White Buildings'* (New York: Liveright, 1972) p. xxxi.
15. J. Unterecker, *Voyager. A Life of Hart Crane* (London: Blond, 1970) p. 378.
16. S. Hazo, *Hart Crane: An Introduction and Interpretation* (New York: Barnes and Noble, 1963) p. 56.
17. Shelley tells his friend Thomas Peacock that homosexuality is 'a subject to be handled with that delicate caution which either I cannot or I will not practise in other matters'. Quoted in Richard Holmes, *Shelley: The Pursuit* (1974; rpt. Harmondsworth: Penguin, 1987) p. 431.
18. *Observer*, 23 July 1989.
19. *Observer*, 21 August 1988.
20. *The Sunday Times*, 3 April 1983.
21. *The Sunday Times*, 27 May 1984.
22. Iris Murdoch, *Sartre: Romantic Realist* (Cambridge: Bowes and Bowes, 1953) pp. 19, 20.
23. Quoted in Mark Lilly, 'Writing Out' in *The Advocate*, 14 August 1982 p. 9.
24. *The Sunday Times*, 24 April 1983.

25. Betty Frieden, *The Feminine Mystique* (1963; rpt. Harmondsworth: Penguin, 1982) pp. 239–40.
26. Ibid., p. 240. Frieden also tells us that gay men are not real men, and hate all women because they feel that it is their excessive and culpable attachment to their mothers that has denied them their virility. She equates 'maturity' and 'manhood' with heterosexuality. The relevant passage speaks of the:

    woman who lives through her son, whose femininity is used in virtual seduction of her son, who attaches her son to her with such dependence that he can never mature to love a woman, nor can he, often, cope as an adult with life on his own. The love of men masks his forbidden excessive love for his mother; his hatred and revulsion for all women is a reaction to the one woman who kept him from becoming a man. (p. 239)

27. R. W. B. Lewis, *The Poetry of Hart Crane. A Critical Study* (Princeton, NJ: Princeton University Press, 1967) p. 196.
28. Ibid., p. 339.
29. Woods, *Articulate Flesh*, pp. 140–1.
30. Valerie Minogue, *Proust: 'Du Côté de chez Swann'* (Arnold: London, 1973) p. 14.
31. Ibid., p. 34.
32. From Marcel Reich-Ranicki, *Thomas Mann and his Family*, quoted in a review by Desmond Christy, *Guardian*, 18 August 1989.
33. Phillip Knightley, 'T. E. Lawrence', in Jeffrey Meyers (ed.), *The Craft of Literary Biography* (London: Macmillan, 1985) p. 164.
34. 'The Phrase Unbearably Repeated', pp. 38–46 in T. B. O'Daniel (ed.), *James Baldwin* (London: Ad Donker, 1977) p. 38.
35. *Observer*, 9 February 1986.
36. Jeffrey Meyers, *Homosexuality and Literature, 1890–1930* (London: Athlone Press, 1977).
37. See, for example, *Hemingway* (1986; rpt. London: Paladin, 1987) p. 89.
38. Jeffrey Meyers, 'Gregory Woods, *Articulate Flesh* (New Haven, Conn.: Yale University Press, 1987)', *Journal of English and Germanic Philology*, vol. 88 (1989) pp. 126–9.
39. Ibid., p. 126.
40. Ibid., p. 127
41. Ibid.
42. Ibid.
43. Ibid., pp. 128–9.
44. It is well to remember that homophobic attitudes are still very strong in the culture generally. Feminist writer Dale Spender can write an essay on women's writing now and not mention lesbians once (*Bookcase*, no. 6, 1984, p. 14). The *West Indian Digest* carries an attack on Lizzie Borden's feminist film *Born in Flames* because of 'strong sympathy with and apparent encouragement of lesbianism'

(no. 103, February 1984, p. 49). The review is written by an anonymous black male.

45. Meyers, *Homosexuality and Literature*, p. 3.
46. Oliver Bernard, *Arthur Rimbaud: Collected Poems* (Harmondsworth: Penguin, 1962) p. xxx.

Notes to Chapter 2

1. Louis Crompton, *Byron and Greek Love* (London: Faber and Faber, 1985).
2. Quoted in William Hazlitt, *The Spirit of the Age* (1825; rpt. London: Collins, 1969) p. 121.
3. *The Picture of Dorian Gray* (1891; rpt. Oxford: Oxford University Press, 1987).
4. See the chapter entitled 'Georgian Homophobia' in Crompton, *Byron and Greek Love*, and *passim*.
5. Walter Gratzer, review of Richard Davenport-Hines, *Sex, Death and Punishment: Attitudes to Sex and Sexuality in Britain since the Renaissance* (Glasgow: Collins, 1990) in *Guardian Weekly*, 10 March 1990, p. 26.
6. Jeffrey Meyers, *Homosexuality and Literature. 1890–1930* (London: Athlone Press, 1977), p. 31.
7. *The Sunday Times*, 24 April 1983.
8. Quoted in Richard Pine, *Oscar Wilde* (Dublin: Gill and Macmillan, 1983) p. 17.
9. *Complete Works of Oscar Wilde* (1948; rpt. London: Collins, 1971), p. 341.
10. Quoted in Pine, *Oscar Wilde*, p. 49.
11. Quoted in ibid., p. 61.
12. Quoted in ibid., p. 67; *Dorian Gray*, p. xxiii.
13. *Dorian Gray*, pp. 6, 18.
14. Ibid., p. 78.
15. Ibid., p. xxiii.

Notes to Chapter 3

1. Quoted in Paul Theroux, *Sunrise with Seamonsters* (Hamish Hamilton: London, 1985) p. 92.
2. This infatuation, as one sometimes feels it is appropriate to describe Cavafy's relationship with Alexandria, is certainly infectious: in literary terms, the best homage to Cavafy's evocation of his city is Laurence Durrell's *Alexandria Quartet*, in which 'the old poet', as Cavafy is called in the work, is constantly alluded to.
3. For example: 'Love is like a flower, it must flower and fade;/if it doesn't fade, it is not a flower, . . .' (D. H. Lawrence, 'The Mess of Love').

4. The rustling of the silk is discontinued,
Dust drifts over the court-yard,
There is no sound of footfall, and the leaves
Scurry into heaps and lie still,
And she the rejoicer of the heart is beneath them:

A wet leaf that clings to the threshold.
('Liu Ch'e ', quoted entire)

Notes to Chapter 4

1. *Maurice* (London: Edward Arnold, 1971).
2. It is interesting to note that the novel's wording here – 'Hall was one of them' – employs exactly the same usage famously employed by Prime Minister Thatcher in the 1980s to indicate close political supporters. The phrase adequately represents a narrowness and inward-looking nature.
3. Forster believed in the greenwood literally, as a place where in this case gay men could physically effect a pastoral escape route. In the terminal note to *Maurice*, he speaks of its literal disappearance:

   Our greenwood ended catastrophically and inevitably. Two great wars demanded and bequeathed regimentation which the public services adopted and extended, science lent her aid, and the wildness of our island, never extensive, was stamped upon and built over and patrolled in no time. There is no forest or fell to escape to today, no cave in which to curl up, no deserted valley for those who wish neither to reform nor corrupt society but to be left alone. (p. 240)

Notes to Chapter 5

1. Paul Fussell, *The Great War and Modern Memory* (London: Oxford University Press, 1975) pp. 279–80.
2. Quoted in Martin Taylor (ed.), *Lads. Love Poetry of the Trenches* (London: Constable, 1989) p. 23.
3. Siegried Sassoon, *Diaries 1915–1918*, edited and introduced by Rupert Hart-Davis (London: Faber, 1983) p. 94.
4. As works of art reflect not only states of mind but literary conventions, it could of course be argued that the excessive ardour evident in the writings under discussion is as much a product of the latter as of the former.
5. In general, effeminate gay men are despised because they are effeminate, that is, like women. The hatred of effeminate men is an aspect of straight men's hatred of women. And women's hatred of effeminate gay men is, on this view, self-hatred.
6. *Sun*, 9 August 1990.

7. Quoted in Richard Holmes, *Shelley. The Pursuit* (1974; rpt. Harmondsworth: Penguin, 1987) p. 433.
8. See note 2 above for bibliographical details. The long introduction is one of the best short studies of the subject available, and I am indebted to it for a number of suggestions. Most of the poems quoted in my chapter are taken from poems included by Taylor in his anthology.
9. W. G. Thomas, 'Ten Years After' (in Taylor, *Lads. Love Poetry of the Trenches*, p. 152).
10. Richard Aldington, 'Reserve' (in ibid., p. 149). In his poem 'Concert', Aldington explores this theme again:

    Am I dead? Withered? Grown old?
    That not the least flush of desire
    Tinges my unmoved flesh,
    And that instead of women's living bodies
    I see dead men – you understand? – dead men . . .
    (in Taylor, p. 197)

11. Robert Nichols, 'The Secret' (in ibid., p. 149).
12. Robert Graves, 'Two Fusiliers' (in ibid., p. 219).
13. Studdert Kennedy, 'Passing the Love of Women' (in ibid., p. 147).
14. George Lewis, 'To My Mate' (in ibid., p. 123).
15. Anon, 'Dicky Boy An' Me' (in ibid., p. 210).
16. Wilfred Owen, 'Disabled' (in ibid., p. 211).
17. Siegfried Sassoon, 'Blighters' (in Brian Gardner (ed.), *Up the Line to Death* (1964; rpt. London: Methuen, 1986) p. 115).
18. E. A. MacIntosh, 'In Memoriam' (in Taylor, *Lads. Love Poetry of the Trenches*, pp. 137–8).
19. E. F. Wilkinson, 'To Leslie' (in ibid., p. 178).
20. Ivor Gurney, 'To His Love' (in ibid., p. 181).
21. 'Diaries', p. 45.
22. Robert Nichols, 'By the Wood' (in Taylor, *Lads. Love Poetry of the Trenches*, p. 192).
23. E. Hilton Young, 'Return' (in ibid., p. 205).
24. Rupert Brooke, 'Peace' (in ibid., p. 66).
25. A. P. Herbert, 'The Bathe' (in ibid., pp. 84–5).
26. Patrick MacGill, 'Red Wine' (in ibid., p. 133).
27. Siegfried Sassoon, 'Prelude: The Troops' (in ibid., p. 87).
28. R. D. Greenway, 'Soldiers Bathing' (in ibid., p. 133).
29. F. S. Woodley, 'To Lieut. O'D' (in ibid., p. 134).
30. Ezra Pound, 'Hugh Selwyn Mauberley' (in ibid., pp. 215–6).
31. Richard Dennys, 'The Question' (in ibid., p. 135).
32. E. F. Wilkinson, 'Memories' (in ibid., p. 125).
33. Wilfred Gibson, 'Lament' (in ibid., p. 218).
34. Edward Shanks, 'Elegy. For J.N., died of wounds, October 1916' (in ibid., p. 180).
35. Siegfried Sassoon, 'Sick Leave' (in ibid., p. 189).

36. E. A. MacIntosh 'From Home. To the men who fell at Beaumont-Hamel' (in ibid., p. 189–90).
37. Wilfred Owen, 'I Saw His Round Mouth's Crimson' (in ibid., p. 91).
38. W. N. Hodgson, 'Glimpse' (in ibid., p. 63).
39. Geoffrey Faber, 'The Modern Achilles' (in ibid., p. 70).
40. Geoffrey Faber, 'Mechanic Repairing a Motor-Cycle' (in ibid., p. 129–30).
41. R. D. Greenway, 'Soldiers Bathing' (in ibid., p. 133).
42. A. P. Herbert, 'The Bathe' (in Taylor, ibid., p. 85).
43. Frank Prewett, 'Voices of Women' (in ibid., p. 145).
44. E. A. MacIntosh, 'In Memoriam' (in ibid., p. 138).
45. Harold Monro, 'Carrion' (in ibid., p. 136).
46. Richard Aldington, 'Soliloquy 1' (in ibid., p. 98).
47. Herbert Read, 'My Company (iii)' (in ibid., p. 98).
48. Siegfried Sassoon, 'Memoirs of an Infantry Officer' (London: Faber, 1930) p. 89.
49. Taylor, *Lads. Love Poetry of the Trenches,* p. 18.
50. Richard Dennys, 'Better Far to Pass Away' (in ibid., p. 67).
51. Now more than ever seems it rich to die,
    To cease upon the midnight with no pain . . .
    (Keats, 'Ode to a Nightingale, stanza vi).

    If it were now to die,
    'Twere now to be most happy; for I fear
    My soul hath her content so absolute
    That not another comfort like to this
    Succeeds in unknown fate.
    (Shakespeare, *Othello,* 11. i. 183–7).

52. Geoffrey Dearmer, 'The Dead Turk' (in Taylor, *Lads. Love Poetry of the Trenches,* p. 166).
53. Charles Carrington, quoted in ibid., p. 157.
54. Robert Nichols, 'Fulfilment' (in ibid., p. 150).
55. Patrick MacGill, 'Matey' (in ibid., p. 111).
56. E. A. MacIntosh, 'In Memoriam. R.M. Stalker' (in ibid., p. 115).
57. Raymond Heywood, 'A Man's Man' (in ibid., p. 175).
58. Studdert Kennedy, 'His Mate' (in ibid., p. 113).
59. Wilfred Gibson, 'Sentry Go' (in ibid., p. 81).
60. Quoted in Dominic Hibberd (ed.), *Wilfred Owen: War Poems and Others* (London: Chatto and Windus, 1973) p. 137.
61. Siegfried Sassoon, 'The Death-Bed' (in Taylor, *Lads. Love Poetry of the Trenches,* p. 101).
62. J. B. Priestley, *Margin Released: A Writer's Reminiscences and Reflections* (London: Heinemann, 1962) p. 89.
63. Edward de Stein, 'Envoie' (in Taylor, *Lads. Love Poetry of the Trenches,* p. 205).

Notes to Chapter 6

1. *The Thief's Journal* (1949; rpt. Harmondsworth: Penguin, 1956); *The Miracle of the Rose* (1951; rpt. Harmondsworth: Penguin, 1975); *Prisoner of Love* (London: Picador, 1989).
2. Jean-Paul Sartre, *Saint Genet: Actor and Martyr*, trans. B. Frechtman (1952; rpt. New York: Pantheon, 1963.)
3. Quoted in T. Eddy, 'Genet's Crimes' in *Siren*, October 1986, p. 29.

Notes to Chapter 7

1. *The Glass Menagerie* (1948; rpt. Harmondsworth: Penguin, 1978); *A Streetcar Named Desire* (1949; rpt. Harmondsworth: Penguin, 1978).
2. *Vieux Carré* (New York: New Directions, 1979).
3. *Small Craft Warnings* (1974; rpt. Harmondsworth: Penguin, 1978).
4. *The Rose Tattoo* (1954; rpt. Harmondsworth: Penguin, 1983) p. 25.
5. *Cat on a Hot Tin Roof* (1956; rpt. Harmondsworth: Penguin, 1981) p. 81.
6. Ibid., p. 79.
7. *A Streetcar Named Desire*, p. 136.
8. *Orpheus Descending* (1955; rpt. Harmondsworth: Penguin, 1983) p. 280.
9. Ibid., p. 273.
10. Ibid., p. 313.
11. Ibid., p. 314.
12. *The Rose Tattoo*, p. 27.
13. Ibid., p. 44.
14. *Sweet Bird of Youth* (1962; rpt. Harmondsworth: Penguin, 1978) p. 47.
15. *The Rose Tattoo*, p. 45.
16. Ibid., p. 45.
17. Ibid., p. 25.
18. *Sweet Bird of Youth*, p. 63.
19. Ibid., p. 20.
20. Ibid., p. 36.
21. Ibid., p. 41.
22. Ibid., p. 41.
23. Ibid., p. 42.
24. Ibid., p. 47.
25. Ibid., p. 48.
26. Foreword to *Sweet Bird of Youth*, p. 10.

Notes to Chapter 8

1. *Confessions of a Mask* (1949; rpt. London: Panther, 1972).
2. *Sun and Steel* (1968; trans. J. Bester, London: Secker and Warburg, 1971).

3. Henry Scott Stokes, *The Life and Death of Yukio Mishima* (London: Owen, 1975) p. 248.
4. Quoted in Stokes, *Life and Death of Yukio Mishima*. p. 64.
5. Quoted in ibid., p. 224.
6. Quoted in ibid., p. 203.
7. Quoted in ibid., pp. 163–4.
8. Quoted in ibid., pp. 199–200.
9. Quoted in ibid., p. 249.
10. *Patriotism* in *Death in Midsummer and Other Stories* (London: New Directions, 1966) pp. 114–15.
11. *Sun and Steel*, pp. 28–9.
12. Catalogue to the Tobu Exhibition, quoted in Stokes, *Life and Death of Yukio Mishima*, p. 184.
13. *Sun and Steel*, pp. 27–8.
14. Ibid., p. 39.
15. Ruth Benedict, *The Chrysanthemum and the Sword* (London: Routledge and Kegan Paul, 1967).
16. Quoted in Stokes, *Life and Death of Yukio Mishima*, p. 227.
17. *The Times*, 24 September 1969.
18. *Queen*, January 1970, pp. 40–42.
19. *Sun and Steel*, pp. 57–9.
20. Quoted in Stokes, *Life and Death of Yukio Mishima*, p. 193.

Notes to Chapter 9

1. *Another Country* (1962; rpt. London: Black Swan, 1987).*Giovanni's Room* (1956; rpt. London: Black Swan, 1984).
2. Donald B. Gibson, 'James Baldwin: The Political Anatomy of Space', in T. B. O'Daniel (ed.), *James Baldwin. A Critical Evaluation* (London: Ad Donker, 1977) pp.12–13.
3. John Lash, 'Baldwin Beside Himself: A Study in Modern Phallicism', in T. B. O'Daniel, *James Baldwin*, p. 52.
4. Willy Loman in *Death of a Salesman*, and Keller in *All My Sons* surrender nothing less than their integrity and humanity, in exchange for family prestige and the respect of a fly-blown yahoo culture.
5. Gore Vidal, *Pink Triangle and Yellow Star* (London: Granada, 1983).
6. This fear of 'tainting' is widespread. When I served on the executive of the National Council for Civil Liberties in the early 1980s, we regularly received letters saying that lesbian/gay rights were giving civil liberties a bad name. Far-left revolutionary groups in the United Kingdom have only recently (some have not done so) abandoned their notion that homosexuality is a ruling class pathology, and that there are no working class gays. The Labour Party is still homophobic, sometimes more so than the Conservatives, and its brief period of token espousal of gay rights has long been considered too expensive in electoral terms.

7. Most oppressed groups find themselves opposed to other such groups rather than their (rationally considered) natural enemies. For example, the way successive British Governments managed to set Protestants against Catholics in Northern Ireland, when each group had genuine grievances against that Government, was extraordinarily skilful. In today's Britain, the success of the popular press in turning their working-class readers against trade unionists, Irish nationalists, feminists, foreigners and so on, is an equally dramatic example. In America, Chicano gangs fight Puerto Ricans who fight Hispanics – and the rich of Beverley Hills and Washington and the garden suburbs, the people who run America, just read about it in the paper and get another guard dog.

   On the political stage, of course, Baldwin was not afraid of being partisan and his essays and speeches and actions in the very streets demonstrated a commitment to the struggle for racial equality; for this very reason, precisely because he was as it were in the front line of political activity, his intellectual and emotional honesty in fiction is so impressive.
8. Heinz Heger, *The Men with the Pink Triangle* (Gay Men's Press: London, 1980).

Notes to Chapter 10

1. In his study of Orton's life and work: John Lahr, *Prick Up Your Ears* (London: Allen Lane, 1978).
2. Simon Shepherd, *Because We're Queers* (London: GMP, 1989).
3. Quoted in Joe Orton, *The Complete Plays* (London: Methuen, 1976) p. 20.
4. *The Erpingham Camp* in *The Complete Plays*, p. 279.
5. *The Ruffian on the Stair* in *The Complete Plays*, p. 33.
6. *Funeral Games* in *The Complete Plays*, p. 333.
7. Ibid., p. 335.
8. *The Ruffian on the Stair* in *The Complete Plays*, p. 57.
9. '. . . it is a tale/Told by an idiot, full of sound and fury,/Signifying nothing' (*Macbeth*, V. v. 26–8).
10. *Funeral Games* in *The Complete Plays*, p. 326.
11. *The Ruffian on the Stair* in *The Complete Plays*, p. 31.
12. *What the Butler Saw* in *The Complete Plays*, p. 397.
13. Matthew XXV, 26–30 (New International Version).
14. *The Good and Faithful Servant* in *The Complete Plays*, p. 153.

Notes to Chapter 11

1. Christopher Isherwood, *A Single Man* (1964; rpt. Harmondsworth: Penguin, 1969).
2. Ibid.
3. Even factually; it refers to George's death, whereas in the novel it is ambiguous.

4. This is common enough. Peregrine Worsthorne, one of Fleet Street's most vitriolic homophobes, revealed in a recent *Daily Telegraph* reminiscence that he had been seduced as a boy by the (now) singer George Melly.
5. Erich Fromm, *The Fear of Freedom* (1942; rpt. London: Ark, 1985) p. 23.

Notes to Chapter 12

1. Andrew Holleran, *Dancer from the Dance* (1978; rpt. London: Corgi, 1980).
2. For example, Tom Wingfield's speech as narrator in Scene 5 of *The Glass Menagerie*:

   > Adventure and change were imminent in this year. They were waiting around the corner for all these kids.
   > Suspended in the mist over Berchtesgaden, caught in the folds of Chamberlain's umbrella –
   > In Spain there was Guernica!
   > But here there was only hot swing music and liquor, dance halls, bars, and movies, and sex that hung in the gloom like a chandelier and flooded the world with brief, deceptive rainbows. . . . (Tennessee Williams, *The Glass Menagerie* (1948; rpt. Harmondsworth: Penguin, 1978) p. 265)

3. In a technically 'stricter' age, the Russian's characters look to duty, to work, to idealistic schemes like forestation, as well as to illicit love.
4. Andrew Holleran, *Nights in Aruba* (1983; rpt. Plume: New York, 1984).

Notes to Chapter 13

1. *The Lost Language of Cranes* (1986; rpt. Harmondsworth: Penguin, 1988).
2. An expression I owe to Greg Woods.
3. *The Fire Next Time* (London: Michael Joseph, 1963).
4. From *The Old Cumberland Beggar*.
5. If this degree of enslavement to received and tyrannical public opinion seems exaggerated in the novel, I should say that I know a man whose parents love him very much but they are prepared entirely to forego seeing him because they cannot adequately or convincingly explain to the next-door neighbours the status of the boyfriend who accompanies their son to the house. They would rather not see their son than acknowledge his sexuality to relative strangers whose standards and character they do not necessarily respect.

Index